THE EROSION OF AUTONOMY IN LONG-TERM CARE

THE EROSION OF AUTONOMY IN LONG-TERM CARE

Charles W. Lidz
Lynn Fischer
Robert M. Arnold

New York Oxford
OXFORD UNIVERSITY PRESS
1992

Oxford University Press

Oxford New York Toronto
Delhi Bombay Calcutta Madras Karachi
Kuala Lumpur Singapore Hong Kong Tokyo
Nairobi Dar es Salaam Cape Town
Melbourne Auckland

and associated companies in
Berlin Ibadan

Published by Oxford University Press, Inc.,
200 Madison Avenue, New York, New York 10016

Library of Congress Cataloging-in-Publication Data
Lidz, Charles W.
The erosion of autonomy in long-term care / Charles W. Lidz, Lynn Fischer, Robert M. Arnold.
p. cm. Includes bibliographical references and index.
ISBN 0-19-507394-0
1. Nursing home patients—United States. 2. Autonomy (Psychology) in old age. 3. Aged—Long-term care. I. Fischer, Lynn, 1956–. II. Arnold, Robert M., 1957–. III. Title. IV. Title: Erosion of autonomy in long term care.
[DNLM: 1. Homes for the Aged—United States. 2. Interpersonal Relations. 3. Long-Term Care—in old age. 4. Nursing Homes—in old age—United States. 5. Patient Advocacy. WT 30 L715e]
RA997.L54 1992 362.1′6—dc20
DNLM/DLC
for Library of Congress 92-6085

9 8 7 6 5 4 3 2 1

Printed in the United States of America
on acid-free paper

C.W.L.
To my wife, Lynn

L.F.
To my grandmother, Edith Gertrude Baker

R.M.A.
To my parents,
Stan Arnold and Joan Huber

Preface

As a nation, America is committed to autonomy. The individual is so deeply revered in our political rhetoric that it sometimes seems to consume our concerns for other important goals. Yet it is hardly a secret that our practice rarely lives up to our aspirations. The treatment and behavior of those individuals who are institutionalized for long periods of time: prisoners, mental patients in long-term hospitals, and the disabled elderly in nursing homes bear witness to caretaking's failure.

In the last two decades, autonomy of patients has also become the major focus of debate in medical ethics. In a wide variety of different medical contexts, ethicists have argued forcefully that routine practices in medicine do not pay sufficient deference to patient autonomy. This volume is grounded in the medical ethics debates about autonomy and seeks to extend that perspective to nursing home care for the elderly. The fundamental issue is what might be done to improve the autonomy of the elderly in long-term care institutions.

In order to find an answer to this problem, we undertook a participant observation study of two nursing home units and an "independent living" facility. The results strongly suggest that the view of how to promote patient autonomy that is prevalent in medical ethics will not be very helpful in long-term care settings. As a result, we have had to rethink what autonomy means and how it might be framed so that it would be a useful conceptual tool for helping those who must spend their last years in nursing homes.

Equally important, we have tried in this volume to provide a clear picture of *how* the routine practices of nursing homes interfere with patient autonomy. These routine practices, of course, reflect other values that are important to us all, such as preserving the patients' physical health and providing care efficiently and at a low cost. It is not our goal to specify which values are most important. However, we have sought to describe just which values and practices interfere with the patients' ability to direct their own lives to the greatest extent to which they are able.

Finally, by describing the ways in which many of the same issues that appear to impede patient autonomy are dealt with in an independent living setting, we have sought to lay out an alternative way of providing long-term care for the disabled elderly that supports a more autonomous lifestyle.

Pittsburgh, Pennsylvania
June 1992

C.W.L.
L.F.
R.M.A.

Acknowledgments

The work on this book began with a telephone call to Chuck Lidz from Ye-fan Wang Glavin, PhD, then an NIMH postdoctoral fellow in the Department of Psychiatry at The University of Pittsburgh. Dr. Glavin was interested in nursing home care for the elderly and knew of Lidz's interest in ethical issues surrounding autonomy. She excitedly reported that the Retirement Research Foundation had started an initiative to develop ways to improve autonomy among nursing home residents. With the advice and counsel of Alan Meisel, JD, the Director of the Center for Medical Ethics at the University, they developed a proposal much like we started with in this study. However, by the time the study began, Dr Glavin had left the city for a new position and it became necessary to build a new team.

The key member of this new team was Lynn Fischer. An experienced ethnographer, she and Lidz had worked together before and they shared an understanding about how the work needed to be done. We also recruited Steven Jarvis, MD, a postdoctoral fellow in the same program with Dr Glavin. Dr Jarvis had a long-standing interest in health care for the elderly and was eager to learn field work methods, and he signed on to do some of the observation. Joanne Best, RN, joined the group and provided us with consistently well focused advice about practical issues in nursing home care. Once data collection was complete, Bob Arnold become involved. He quickly began to reformulate the ethical and social scientific analysis. Jason Baim played a significant role in the design and implementation of the coding system.

A grant from the Retirement Research Foundation involved more than simply completing the proposed research. Under the very active direction of Foundation Vice-President Brian Hofland, all the grantees met twice each year for two days. What initially seemed like an unwanted chore turned into a fascinating opportunity to learn from others in the field. Useful input came from Christine Cassel, MD, Nancy Dubler, LLB, Margaret Gatz, PhD, and many others. Particularly helpful were Rosalie Kane, DSW, whose wide grasp of the issues in this field may be without parallel, and George Agich, PhD, whose fascinating phenomenological framing of the issues had a major impact on our work.

Brian Hofland also helped the direction of this work by strongly suggesting that we should constitute a group of advisors. With his advice we choose Rosalie Kane, DSW, Jaber Gubrium, PhD, Louis Burgio, PhD, and H.R. (Rick) Moody, PhD. Their breadth of experience and understanding of the larger issues in long-term care were invaluable in the eventual framing of this report.

We are indebted to all of these people, but most of all to the staff and residents of the study site, which we simply refer to as "the facility." They were patient with us and, in several cases, spent long hours with us reviewing the workings of the facility and their understanding of its strengths and weaknesses. We hope that this work justifies their time and trust.

We also want to thank the staffs of the University of Pittsburgh Center for Medical Ethics and the Law and Psychiatry Program of the Department of Psychiatry who put up with us through the many trials and tribulations of this work.

Contents

THE EROSION OF AUTONOMY IN LONG-TERM CARE

1

The Meaning of Autonomy in Long-Term Care

Over the last fifteen years, health care ethicists have focused increasingly on the notion of autonomy. Until the 1960s the dominant (and perhaps only) values in discussions of health care ethics were beneficence and nonmaleficence. The Hippocratic Oath succinctly summarizes this view, enjoining physicians "to help or at least to do no harm." Professionals were to restore the patient's health or, if this was not possible, at least to prevent further pain, suffering, or disability. This view of ethics required health care professionals to promote the patient's best interest as interpreted from the health care professional's perspective. According to this view, the job of professionals is to use their knowledge to weigh the costs and benefits of available therapies and to determine which treatments are in the patient's "best interests." Beneficence required professionals to act in accordance with their expert judgments, rather than making decisions based on the patient's assessment of what is in her best interest. In nursing homes this leads to an emphasis on the individual's physical well-being.

This conception of ethics dictates a certain model of professional-patient relationship. Generally speaking, professionals prescribe and patients comply. Patients go to the doctor because they suspect they are ill, are assessed by their doctor, are told what is wrong with them and what they need to do in order to get better, and then are expected to follow the doctor's orders (Parsons 1951).

In the last two decades, a new value has been introduced into the discussion of health care ethics—patient autonomy (Whitbeck 1985). In contrast to beneficence, autonomy requires health care providers to follow the patient's wishes, rather than their own determination of what is best for the patient. In the United States, respect for autonomy first emerged as a central concern in research ethics. In response to Nazi use of unconsenting humans in experimentation to advance the goals of science[1], the Nuremberg Code established the primary role of autonomy in human experimentation. The limiting factor that determines whether an individual becomes a research subject is the subject's voluntary, informed consent, rather than just a scientist's belief that research will yield important results.

The doctrine of informed consent also has become a (if not the) central theme of health care ethics (Faden and Beauchamp 1986). The theoretical justification of informed consent has relied heavily on the notion of autonomy. To seek the patient's permission prior to instituting treatment shows respect for the patient's autonomy by acknowledging that the patient makes the final decision regarding a therapeutic plan. The following quote from a famous court case concerning informed consent, *Nathanson v Kline*, makes this connection clear:

> Anglo-American law starts with the premise of thoroughgoing self-determination. It follows that each man is considered to be master of his own body, and he may, if he be of sound mind, expressly prohibit the performance of life saving surgery, or other medical treatment. A doctor may well believe that an operation or other form of treatment is desirable or necessary but the law does not permit him to substitute his own judgment for that of the patient (*Nathanson v Kline* 1960).

Respecting autonomy in health care is thought to be important for two reasons (Cassel, Hofland unpublished; Cassell 1989; Childress 1982; Collopy 1986; President's Commission 1982). First, respecting autonomy is valuable because of its likely consequences. Contrary to the conception of well being found in the Hippocratic Oath, allowing people to make their own choices generally is felt to result in maximizing the patients' best interests (Sartorius 1983). This is the traditional liberal argument that persons are usually better judges of their best interests than others, even benevolent others. Best interests is not an objectively determined, unified notion. What is in a person's best interest can be defined only in the context of that particular person's goals and values. Although a particular professional's conception of health may be in most patients' best interest, this is not always so. Elderly patients may feel that promoting health is not as important to them as other goals such as staying comfortable or spending time engaged in other pursuits. Even when a health care goal is undisputed, a variety of approaches may be available; which option is best for a particular individual may depend on the impact of the different approaches on the individual's nonmedical goals. Given the subjective nature of one's "best interest," most ethicists feel that the persons whose interests are at stake are best qualified to make decisions regarding themselves.

More is involved in respecting autonomy than its instrumental value (Dworkin 1989). One can imagine situations in which an external expert could know better than an individual what was in her best interest, but even in those situations many philosophers would argue that autonomous decision-making by the patient is still preferable. There is an intrinsic good to be gained from allowing an individual to direct her own life (Kant 1964). Subjectively we often experience the same sense of desire for autonomy. This is manifested in a preference for being an instrument of one's own plans and desires rather than to have one's life determined by others. A person wants to have the sense of defining her own values and deciding how to act to achieve her goals even if these decisions are sometimes incorrect.[2]

Although it may be clear why autonomy is important in making health care decisions, it is far from clear what the term means. Autonomy is derived from the Greek *autos* (self) and *nomos* (rule or governance or law), and was first used to refer to self-rule in Greek city states. The ambiguity of the term is clear from the diversity of definition that we find among the leading authorities. For example, the President's Commission defines autonomy or self-determination as "an individual's exercise of the capacity to form, revise and pursue personal plans for life" (President's Commission 1982); Beauchamp and Childress define autonomy as "being one's own person, without constraint either by another's action or by psychological or physical limitations" (Beauchamp, Childress 1989); Rawls characterizes acting autonomously as "acting from principles that we would consent to as a free and equal rational being" (Rawls 1971); Lucas says "I, and I alone, am ultimately responsible for the decisions I make and am in that sense autonomous" (Lucas 1966); while recent theorists such as Gerald Dworkin and George Agich have characterized autonomy as the ability to identify with the decisions that one makes (Dworkin 1989, Agich 1988). Other theorists, such as Collopy and Thomasma, define autonomy not as a unitary concept but as a group of related notions (Collopy 1988, Thomasma 1984).

It is apparent that autonomy is being used in a very broad way. As Gerald Dworkin points out:

> It is equated with dignity, integrity, individuality, independence, responsibility, and self-knowledge. It is identified with qualities of self-assertion, with critical reflection, with freedom from obligation, with absence of external causation, with knowledge of one's own interests. It is even equated by some economists with the impossibility of interpersonal comparisons. It is related to actions, to beliefs, to reasons for acting, to rules, to the will of other

> persons, to thoughts, and to principles. About the only features held constant from one author to another are that autonomy is a feature of persons and that it is a desirable quality to have (Dworkin 1989:6).

The lack of clarity regarding what is meant when one refers to autonomy has hampered the use of the term in both moral discourse and the development of health care policy. As long as the meaning of autonomy is unclear, it is unlikely that the concept will be applied in a consistent manner. Moreover, confusion regarding what is meant by autonomy results in its being used to justify contradictory positions. For example, some might argue that a hemiplegic patient's refusal to attend occupational therapy classes in the nursing home should be honored because it respects her autonomy, while others might argue that forcing her to go to therapy will increase her function and therefore increase her autonomy. If the different concepts of autonomy are clarified, we will have a better understanding of exactly what we are trying to respect.

In assessing different concepts of autonomy we need to be aware that there are a variety of different purposes for which scholars have defined autonomy (Christman 1989). Some have sought to define a theory of autonomy for the purposes of exploring different systems of governance. In health care ethics, conceptions of autonomy are used to delineate patients' rights to make health care decisions for themselves. The definitions of autonomy are used to delineate who can make such decisions (competence) and what health care professionals must do to respect autonomy (informed consent).

Our task here is somewhat different. We are concerned with improving the autonomy of the elderly living in a long-term care situation. We are concerned with an individual's life situation rather than an individual decision, with the effect of an entire system of care as opposed to a single discussion between professional and patient. Thus, we will find useful different facets of autonomy than would someone concerned with the doctrine of informed consent (Agich 1988, Moody 1988, Whitbeck 1985). Our goal is to explore conceptions of autonomy that both make sense out of the notion that our beliefs, actions, and lives should be our own, and are also useful to the analysis of the impact of social institutions.

Prior to describing the different concepts of autonomy, we need to highlight a common misconception. Many philosophers conceptualize autonomy as being synonymous with independence from external influences; to be autonomous means one is radically self-sufficient, dependent on no one else. Autonomous persons are independent, self-ruled entities who make decisions based solely on their own reasons (Lucas 1966, Wolff 1970; for a critique of this view in the philosophical literature see Agich 1988, Dworkin 1989). Indeed, such a concept might seem to be nothing but an elaboration of the concept of self-direction. What could be more desirable than such total freedom?

Appealing and clear as such a conception of autonomy is, we cannot disagree too strongly with this atomistic context. All human life takes place in a historical, social, and cultural context (Feinberg 1986). One's values and actions are necessarily affected by one's past and environment. No person autonomously chooses her genetic background, her parents, the time period or society in which she was born, or much of her early upbringing. All of these factors place limits on the persons we are and will become and make the notion of an independent, self-ruled person unrealistic. Dworkin summarizes this objection, saying:

> We all know that persons have a history. They develop socially and psychologically in a given environment with a given set of biological endowments. They mature slowly and are heavily influenced by their parents, siblings, peers and culture. What sense does it make to speak of convictions, motivations, principles, and so forth as "self-selected"? This presupposes a notion of self as isolated from the influences just enumerated and what is almost as foolish, that the self which chooses does so arbitrarily. . . . We can no more choose *ab initio* than we can jump out of our skin. To insist on this position is to make autonomy impossible (Dworkin 1989).

A moment's thought will make it clear that such narcissistic self-absorption is not an ideal to that most of us would aspire. It makes it difficult to justify and enforce simple elements of socially acceptable behavior that we teach children, such as sharing, taking turns, and politeness.

Instead of equating autonomy with absolute independence, we will look at more complicated notions of autonomy that recognize that individuals are socially and historically situated. Concepts such as distinctiveness, consistency, understanding, identification, and initiative are likely to be more fruitful than total self-rule in explicating what it means to be autonomous. Rather than asking whether a choice was influenced by others, we will be concerned with how those influences affected the choices and whether the influences subverted the individual's control, reasoning process, or identification.

Different Concepts of Autonomy

There are a number of different views of autonomy that might be helpful in a study such as this. In this section we will outline several of them.

Autonomy as Free Action

Autonomy as free action means that the act is both voluntary and intentional (Miller 1981). An act is intentional if it is willed according to a plan. Intentional acts are not events that merely happen to people. Faden and Beauchamp describe an intentional act this way; "Whether a given act, X, is intentional, depends on whether in performing X the actor could upon reflection say, 'I did X as I planned' and in that sense, 'I did the "X" I intended to do' " (Faden and Beauchamp 1986:243).[3]

Intentional actions are different from those that happen accidentally. If while intending to drink lemonade someone mistakenly drinks a glass of arsenic, it cannot be claimed that she intended to kill herself. Other candidates for unintentional actions include those that are done inadvertently, certain habitual actions such as tics, and actions that are the result of physical force exerted by someone else.

As we noted above, autonomy as free action must be voluntary as well as intentional. A person must be able to say that she did the act because she wanted to rather than because other forces unduly pressured her. What constitutes undue pressure? Faden and Beauchamp address the question by examining the polar extremes of completely voluntary and involuntary acts (Faden and Beauchamp 1986; for a different view see Sartorius 1983). A nonvoluntary act is one in that the person is completely dominated by an external agent. A voluntary act is one that either has not been the target of an influence attempt or, if it has been the target of attempt at influence, was either not successful or did not deprive the actor in any way of willing what she wished to do or believe. Notice that this definition of voluntariness does not exclude all external pressures.[4] A person can be influenced without rendering an action involuntary if the person acts on the basis of what she wants rather than on the basis of an external agent's will.

The problem is determining the effect of various influences on whether an action is one's own and its implications for voluntariness. Although completely voluntary or involuntary actions occur, most actions fall somewhere in between these two extremes. A continuum exists between voluntary and involuntary acts and, correspondingly, between autonomous and nonautonomous acts. In reality, an action may be more or less influenced.

Many authors delineate three groups of external influences. At one extreme are *coercive* influences. By presenting a threat of unwanted and unavoidable harm that a person will be unable to resist, the coercer gains control over another's actions. These influences render the action involuntary and hence nonautonomous. For example, threatening to tie patients into a geri-chair if they do not participate in music therapy probably renders that participation involuntary. At the other extreme are *persuasive* influences. These influences attempt to influence a decision by appealing to reason and, in the final analysis, still leave the decision in the hand of the actor. A patient can, after hearing the reasons for attending music therapy, freely decide to accept or reject the persuader's line of argument. Because these influences do not control another's action they do not impede voluntariness or autonomy.

Between these extremes are a large group of influences that Faden and Beauchamp define as *manipulative*. Manipulative influences are attempts at "noncoercively altering the actual choices available to the person or nonpersuasively altering the person's perception of those choices" (Faden and Beauchamp 1986:261). Manipulative influences have varying effects on the voluntariness of an act. There is no hard-and-fast line between those manipulative influences that substantially interfere with voluntariness (and render a choice nonautonomous) and those that do not.[5]

We have been discussing external forces which render one's actions less than fully autonomous. While it is not our primary interest, it should be noted that forces internal to an individual may also decrease the voluntariness of one's action (Christman 1987; Duggan and Gert 1967). For example, someone who is claustrophobic may want to go into an elevator, but be unable to do so. Addictions and severe compulsions may also control a person so that her behavior no longer reflects the person.[6] We generally characterize this behavior as involuntary, saying "I couldn't help myself."

There is something plausible in this conception of autonomy. It seems to explain our intuition that most of our daily, mundane activities are, in a certain sense, autonomous. Getting out of bed in the morning and wearing black rather than brown shoes are activities that we intend and that are voluntarily chosen. This concept also accounts for our view that most people have at least some capacity for autonomous action. The requirements for autonomy as free action are minimal. As long as one has the ability to form preferences and a sense of self that includes the belief that her actions can influence the environment in predictable ways, one has the capacity to act autonomously. Even very young children and moderately demented individuals are likely to have sufficient capacity to act autonomously, at least most of the time, according to this definition. For example, if, when hungry, a moderately demented patient calls out to be taken to the dining room, we have adequate behavioral grounds for concluding, according to this definition, that this is an autonomous act.

In spite of its inherent plausibility, this concept of autonomy is of limited use for our goal of assessing the effects of institutional structures on autonomy in long-term care. The suggestion that autonomy can be promoted by minimizing pressures on patients about what to do is of little help in a setting like a nursing home in which living up to standards of care (both internally generated standards and those imposed by regulation) requires that staff often pressure some patients to do what they might otherwise not do.

Autonomy as Effective Deliberation

Effective deliberation consists of making a decision based on an understanding of the situation and the possible alternative courses of action (Faden and Beauchamp 1986, Miller 1981). This sense of autonomy is distinct from autonomy as free action. A person can act voluntarily and intentionally without effective deliberation, e.g., when acting impulsively or without an understanding of the consequences of an action. Autonomy as effective deliberation emphasizes acting based on an understanding of the situation, the action, and its consequences, as well as the possible alternatives.

What do we mean by "understanding an act"? Faden and Beauchamp offer the following definition:

> A person has a full or complete understanding of an action if there is a fully adequate apprehension of all the relevant propositions or statements (those that contribute in any way to obtaining an appreciation of the situation) that correctly describe (1) the nature of the action and (2) the foreseeable consequences and possible outcomes that might follow as a result of performing and not performing the action (Faden and Beauchamp 1986).

This definition is obviously only an ideal. Most of our decisions are not made with perfect understanding and, thus, are not perfectly autonomous. The extent to which someone understands an action will depend on the complexity of the decision, what one is told about it, what one's preconceptions were before considering the issues, one's mental capacities at the time, the amount of time one has to analyze the problem, and other situational variables. A decision that is made hurriedly, with limited information and under some stress, is likely to be less fully considered than one made after careful analysis. As with autonomy as free action, this conception of autonomy therefore admits of degrees. The more fully one understands one's action, the alternatives, and their consequences, and makes a decision based on this information, the more autonomous the action is.[7]

There are also different meanings of the term "understand." One meaning of the term is to understand the relevant facts. However, some concepts of "understand" suggest that one must appreciate the implications of these facts for one's life situation. For example, an elderly person who agrees to move to another city to be close to her children may understand that she will leave her friends behind, but may not have considered how lonely she will be without them. The more completely she appreciates the consequences of an action on her life, the more we are inclined to say that she truly understands the situation and, thus, that her decision meets the criteria for autonomy as effective deliberation.

Autonomy as effective deliberation, however, requires more than understanding the facts regarding the situation (Miller 1981). Effective deliberation requires that one's decision be based, in a minimally rational way, on the facts of the situation.[8] Consider, for example, an otherwise healthy 70-year-old woman who says that her primary goal is to live as long as possible. Imagine that this woman develops breast cancer. Even if she understands the risks and benefits of a mastectomy for localized cancer, her refusal of surgery because she is afraid of dying in surgery would be considered the result of noneffective deliberation because she has assigned a nonrational weight to the risk of surgery.

It should be obvious from the above discussion that autonomy as effective deliberation is most relevant when a person is facing a significant decision with clearly identifiable options. It is therefore no surprise that this notion of autonomy has been most extensively relied upon to ground the doctrine of informed consent, particularly for hospitalized patients in need of surgery or some other discrete procedure. In these situations a patient is faced with a decision that has major consequences and risks that the physician describes to the patient. The patient, having acquired this information, can effectively deliberate about what, given her values, she wants to do.

This model is less helpful in thinking about what social structures in the day-to-day life of nursing home patients promote autonomy. Many of these patients have substantial levels of dementia, and demented patients are often limited in their capacity for effective deliberation. Their memory and cognitive processes are often impaired to such a degree that understanding and weighing various options are beyond their capabilities. More importantly, the routine life of long-term care nursing home patients lacks discrete, major decisions with clearly identifiable benefits and costs. Indeed, identifying alternatives and delineating consequences is not the central feature of most of our lives. Most of our daily lives are spent acting in taken-for-granted ways without much explicit analysis of risks and benefits. Life is full of many minor choices—going to music therapy, or watching one TV channel rather than another. We often make decisions based on incomplete information, without consideration of alternatives and without any explicit weighing of costs and benefits. For nursing home patients only the decisions concerning the outside world, e.g., discharge and subsequent placement or selling one's house, constitute problems of the sort in which one might expect autonomy as effective deliberation to be the appropriate standard. Effective deliberation, if it occurs at all, usually occurs regarding unique decisions that have a major impact on a person's life.

Autonomy as Consistency

The above concepts of autonomy focus on isolated, discrete acts. This analysis, while valuable, has limited applicability for our purposes. The analysis of autonomy in long-term care must not focus exclusively on discrete decisions. Instead, it must deal with patterns of living precisely because it is about long-term care. People's lives are not merely a series of individual acts with no connection to one another; human activity is more integrated than this. Autonomous acts are accomplished by people who have a past, present, and future. People have goals and interests that bind activities together in a coordinated way. Individual actions take on added meaning in the context of a person's longer-term goals. Someone whose actions are both free and based on effective deliberation, but who has no longer-term goals, no sense of past or present commitments to call her own, seems more like a computer than an autonomous person. Knowledge of these larger goals may also shed light on the reasons for what appears, given the other criteria, to be less than fully autonomous behavior. For example, a person may not spend time trying to understand everything about a particular decision because, in the scheme of that person's life, the decision is not critically important. Thus, although the decision seemed less autonomous when considered under the criteria for effective deliberation, when one evaluates the act based on knowledge of a person's longer-term concerns, the behavior seems more autonomous.

A different way to think of autonomy is to consider how our actions fit together. Instead of analyzing the autonomy of an action as an isolated unit separated from all other past actions, current involvements, and future directions, we want to understand autonomy in terms of people's long-term goals, current commitments, and past activities (Dworkin 1984, Hayworth 1986). As Ronald Dworkin puts it, "This view of autonomy focuses not on individual decisions one by one, but the place of each decision in a more general program or picture of the life the agent is creating and constructing, a conception of character and achievement that must be allowed its own distinctive integrity" (Dworkin 1984:24).

An analogy may be helpful. Imagine trying to understand sentences or paragraphs in a novel by merely analyzing the constituent words and phrases and their interrelations in isolation from other sentences and paragraphs. Every sentence of the story may be well-written, clean, concise, and reasonable. However, this alone would tell us neither if the story is well-written nor if the characters make sense in light of the rest of the story. To analyze this one would have to determine if the elements of the story made sense in terms of the story line as a whole. The same is true of autonomy. In order to assess whether a particular action is truly an autonomous act requires examining the context in which the act occurs. We have therefore tried to develop a conception of autonomy that takes into consideration this fuller, more integrated sense of a person's life. In this sense, we are taking a novelist's view of an action. It can only be understood in terms of the individual's history, the story in which she currently sees herself involved, and the longer-term direction in which she orients her life.

This integrated notion of autonomy is consistent with the noninstrumental value of autonomy discussed above. As Ronald Dworkin has commented, "This value of autonomy, on this view, lies in the scheme of responsibility it creates; autonomy makes each of us responsible for shaping his own life according to some coherent and distinctive sense of character, conviction and interest" (Dworkin 1984:24).

This approach to autonomy thus assesses the autonomous character of one's life rather than the autonomy of each individual act. This conception seems most relevant to our task—determining the impact of a nursing home setting on the daily lives of the elderly. Life in such a setting, as we shall discuss shortly, is characterized not by major decisions with significant impacts on individuals' lives but by mundane activities that require little or no conscious decision making.

Thus, our final conception of autonomy, autonomy as consistency, emphasizes that the autonomous activity is consistent with an individual's commitments, values, and life plans—i.e., that the person's activities are roughly consistent with the way she views herself. It is an individual's identification with or acceptance of an activity or series of activities that makes an individual act autonomous. Autonomy as consistency places special emphasis on the coherence between the activity in question and the patterns of activity and commitment with which one has been involved, is involved, or plans to be involved over the long term.

There are three basic dimensions of an act's consistency. One is how the action fits in with the person's past activities—roughly that an individual is acting in character (Miller 1981). This concept is exemplified in comments such as "It's just like Mom to not want to go to the dance" or "Dad was always a stubborn guy." One must look at the activities that the individual has engaged in and how enthusiastically or reluctantly she participated, as well as the person's previously stated goals and motivations in order to determine whether or not a decision is autonomous by this standard.

This view of consistency captures our belief that we are more than a random collection of choices and acts. Instead we generally think of a person as an entity that develops within relatively persistent and enduring patterns. The problem with an over-reliance on this one dimension of consistency is that it suggests that a person's self is largely static and does not change over time. A retrospective analysis of autonomy does not allow for autonomous changes in a person's life and direction. One's goals and commitments can change as one ages, gathers new experiences, or finds oneself in different circumstances. However, in spite of its limitations, this retrospective concept of consistency is sometimes the only relevant dimension, particularly with a severely demented patient who can no longer give reasons for what seem to be inconsistent actions. However, a richer conception of autonomy as consistency will take into account one's current views and aspirations.

Thus, we have a second type of consistency, one which views autonomous activities as consistent with current values and commitments. One way of conceptualizing this type of consistency is to focus on the individual's identification with activities. Do I see the activity as consistent with who I am? The more one identifies an activity as one's own, the clearer we are that it is autonomous. As one's identification with activities becomes less positive, they are less clearly one's own and, thus, are less autonomous.

Identification is, however, only a partial understanding of this type of consistency. The term "commitments" refers to the fact that, as a social actor, one is not always completely free to change one's mind. A particular patient may wish to go out for a visit to the mall but feel that she must stay and keep her depressed and lonely friend company. While we might believe that she would be happier if she went to the mall, relationships do involve commitments that we would sometimes rather ignore. Assuming that the relationship was undertaken willingly, actions consistent with those commitments are autonomous and should be honored. Indeed, the absence of such commitments leads to an isolated individual, not an autonomous one.

A final component of autonomy as consistency is consideration of the activity in light of a person's longer-term goals and enterprises.[9] These can vary from specific goals such as learning to play the piano to longer-term, or more encompassing goals such as becoming a better person. Whatever an individual's past or current commitments, human beings usually live at least partially in the future. We have ideas of desirable changes that we try to effectuate, both in our own lives and in those of others about whom we care. Likewise, there are many enduring situations that we try to preserve for the future.

When we speak of autonomy as "self-direction," it is important to remember that a "direction" usually goes somewhere. We need to appreciate the directionality of self-direction. Autonomous activity implies a goal toward which it is directed or an undertaking of which it is a part. Moreover, such a goal does not have to be focused on one's self. Many elderly individuals are deeply committed to working for their churches, their communities, and their families. Assuming such commitments are freely made, they may be important parts of the individuals' autonomous selves. Promoting autonomous activity on their part may not involve promoting their private "best interests," either subjectively or objectively defined.

Of course, an elderly nursing home patient who is weak from a long confinement and whose social relations have deteriorated as her peers have died and her children have moved away may have a limited horizon. She may only plan for the next few weeks as opposed to a younger person who has at least some plans for years ahead. However, that does not limit the importance of the consistency of her action with such longer-term goals.

Whether a particular act is autonomous or not can change depending on one's feeling about an undertaking and its effect on one's self. One's commitment to an enterprise may change, therefore, changing one's assessment of an activity. Ms. Jones, for example, may autonomously undertake to learn to play the piano. However, as she begins to learn how to play she realizes that while she likes the attention she receives from the other residents of the nursing home, she does not like to play the piano. It takes a great deal of time and she finds that she will have to give up other, more enjoyable activities. Soon she wishes that she had never played the piano. However, she continues to play because the other patients request it and cajole her into playing when she expresses reluctance. While she may enter into a contemporaneous commitment one morning to play a recital that afternoon, she clearly cannot be held to the recital that she had planned two months previously. This example shows the complex relationship between an undertaking, self-identity, and autonomy. Ms. Jones' loss of commitment to learning to play the piano changes what started as an autonomous activity into one that is largely nonautonomous.

Of course, consistency cannot stand alone as the only definition of autonomy (Callahan 1984, Collopy 1989, Dworkin 1989, Engelhardt 1989). To begin with, just as effective deliberation does not deal with the relationship of an act to the broader life circumstances of the individual, so consistency does not provide a good way of understanding the autonomous features of the act itself. And, unlike the concept of free action, it says relatively little about the pressures that come to bear on our goals or behavior. Finally, it provides only the loosest of criteria for deciding whether or not a particular act is autonomous. Thus any complete theory of autonomy in the elderly must deal with questions of free action and effective deliberation as well as consistency. However, for our purposes—describing the impact of institutional structures on autonomy—it is a particularly useful framework.

Autonomy, Privacy, and Liberty

While autonomy is an important value in health care, it is not the only value. Privacy and liberty, two concepts closely related to autonomy, are also critical to the evaluation of nursing home structures. A brief review of the relationship between autonomy and these two values will be useful when analyzing the empirical data.

Privacy consists of the ability of an individual to maintain and control access to herself (Beauchamp and Childress 1989, Childress 1982). This access may concern either the physical self or information about the self. Advocates of the right to privacy employ the imagery of concentric circles. In the center is the core self, where an individual's "ultimate secrets—those hopes, fears, and prayers that are beyond sharing with anyone . . ." reside. The next circle consists of intimate secrets about oneself that one shares with one's closest compatriots. Successively larger circles are open to intimate friends, casual acquaintances, and finally all observers. Activities typically interpreted as interfering with privacy include observations of our body, our behavior, or our works without our consent.

Respect for privacy, like respect for autonomy, may become tenuous in nursing homes. De facto, the move from one's own home to a nursing home carries with it a loss of privacy. Privacy is more difficult to respect given the close living quarters and the communal areas for eating, watching television, and talking. The demands of nursing care can also lead to a decreased emphasis on privacy. Our empirical analysis was structured to shed light on how privacy was respected or denied in a nursing home.

Violations of both autonomy and privacy result from a failure to respect an individual as an independent moral agent. Often a violation of one's privacy is also a violation of autonomy, as when a nurse continues to go into a resident's room against her expressed wishes. However, the two concepts are distinct. Autonomy can be interfered with without affecting privacy and vice versa. Consider the following two examples.

- A nurse's aide goes through Mrs. Smith's room without her knowledge.
- A nurse's aide deceives Mrs. Smith into going to music therapy by telling her that her friends will be there.

In the first example, Mrs. Smith's privacy has been violated. Her ability to be self-determining, to be autonomous in her values, decisions, or actions, however, may not have been significantly affected. In the second case, Mrs. Smith's autonomy has been interfered with but her privacy has not been affected. While the aide has affected Mrs. Smith's decision-making, and thus her autonomy, the aide has not learned anything new that Mrs. Smith wished to conceal from her.

It is important to distinguish between these two concepts. Even when a nursing home is unable to promote autonomy, it may still be able to structure care to respect patients' privacy. This is particularly important in the care of moderately demented patients. Thus, in our empirical analysis we will distinguish between violations of privacy and those of autonomy.

Liberty is another concept that is closely related to autonomy. Liberty can be conceptualized as the number of "open options" one has. Feinberg defines an open option as "when I am permitted to do X and I am also permitted to do not-X (that is, to omit doing X), so that it is up to me entirely whether I do X or not" (Feinberg 1984:207). An analogy will make this perspective clearer:

> We can think of life as a kind of maze of railroad tracks connected and disjoined, here and there, by switches. Whenever there is an unlocked switch, which can be pulled one way or the other, there is an "open option"; whenever the switch is locked in one position the other option is "closed." As we chug along our various tracks in the maze, other persons are busily locking and unlocking, opening and closing switches, thereby enlarging and restricting our various movements (Feinberg 1986).[10]

Liberty is an important good in human life. Our interest in having at least a minimum amount of liberty (or open options) is perhaps the easiest to explain. Suppose one's life is totally arranged, ie, all tracks but one are closed, in such a way that all of one's desires and other interests are satisfied. Such a person would nonetheless be lacking many of the attributes critical to human happiness. Her life would approximate that of a robot with no responsibility for her actions, no sense of self-esteem or dignity. There would no longer be any point to changing one's mind, of developing new interests, or of guiding the pursuit of old interests into new channels. "The self-monitoring and self-critical capacities, so essential to human nature, might as well dry up and wither; they would no longer have any function" (Feinberg 1984:211–212).

Up to a certain point, greater amounts of liberty are, like health or economic wealth, generally valued. Feinberg offers three reasons why liberty has value (Feinberg 1986). First, people have an interest in surplus liberty as a hedge against an uncertain future. Having a large number of open options allows people to have the security of knowing that if their interests change and they decide to take a different track, there are alternatives open to them. Second, there is an aesthetic desire to live in a world that presents numerous options, even though they may never be taken up. The symbolic value here is analogous to preferring a bookstore with more books than one could possibly want to read over a more limited one. Finally, and most importantly, liberty creates space for experimentation. Only by testing various paths can one decide what kind of life best suits one's talents, needs, and desires. Without open options one's path is laid out by fate or by others. There is reason to believe, however, that others will not be as sensitive to a person's needs and talents as the person herself.

On the other hand, there is reason to believe that there are limits to the amount of liberty we find helpful. To begin with, there is considerable evidence from cognitive psychology that, faced with a large variety of choices, we quickly work to reduce the choices so as to simplify the decision-making process (Kahneman and Tversky 1982). Second, anomie theorists starting with Durkheim have shown fairly well that insufficient structure in our lives is at least as hard to live with as too much structure (Durkheim 1951).

Liberty may be especially important for nursing home patients. Their physical and mental disabilities already place restrictions on the options open to them. Moreover, the move into a nursing home itself is often seen as closing off many previously open options. For many patients, the nursing home is the area in which they eat, sleep, engage in recreational activities, and visit friends. The number of open and closed options in this environment therefore has an important effect on the amount of liberty a nursing home patient experiences. Nursing homes may limit residents' freedom by regulations that decrease their ability to regulate relatively mundane aspects of their lives, like when to eat or sleep or visit with their neighbors. On the other hand, nursing homes can take steps to help overcome individuals' internal restraints by offering physical therapy and rehabilitation.

Not only is liberty important, in and of itself, it is integral to promoting an individual's autonomy (Hayworth 1986). Liberty and autonomy, while distinct, are closely related concepts. While delineating the options available to a person and whether they are open or closed describes one's liberty, autonomy concerns whether one's choices are one's own. Typically, interference with one's liberty also violates one's autonomy. If a resident is forced to go to physical therapy, not only is this a direct interference with liberty but also a violation of the patient's ability to choose for herself the kind of therapy she wants (or whether she wants any therapy at all). Conversely, assume that a bedridden patient wants to buy her sister a birthday present. By supplying a wheelchair and a van to get her to a shopping area, the nursing home both opens a previously closed option and respects the patient's autonomous choice. Thus, Dworkin concludes that "Liberty . . . [while] not the same as autonomy, [is a] necessary condition for individuals to develop their own aims and interests and to make values effective in the living of their lives" (Dworkin 1989).

The relationship between liberty and autonomy is often more subtle than described above. Increasing the number of open options will not, in and of itself, necessarily increase one's autonomy. If the nursing home does not offer access to the facilities that are necessary for one's chosen undertaking, it does not matter, as far as autonomy is concerned, how many other choices are provided. It does not allow the actualization of one's autonomous choices. To quote Agich:

> [E]ven when individuals are afforded choices, autonomy may not be significantly enhanced because the choice available may not be meaningful for the individuals involved. Ideally, choice that enhances autonomy is choice that is meaningful for individuals and allows them to express and develop their own individuality. If such is not the case, then the true sense of autonomy of persons is not enhanced (Agich 1988:126).

Liberty, while not synonymous with autonomy, is thus an important value in nursing homes. Our empirical study, therefore, pays close attention to the ways in which nursing home regulations and health care professionals limited or expanded the liberty of individuals.

Conclusion

There can be little in the way of autonomous activity if the minimal criterion of free action is not respected. Whatever else autonomy may be, it requires that the activity be intentional and free from coercion. Moreover, it is equally clear that some criterion of understanding and deliberation is necessary for a discrete autonomous act. We do not propose that autonomy as consistency should replace these criteria, but that it is an important supplement for the issues that we are concerned with in this volume.

These three different notions have important implications for determining what it means to respect and promote autonomy in long-term care. If autonomy is conceptualized as free action, one's obligations are largely negative. All that is required is that the health care professional not interfere with the patient's decision-making. Non-interference, then, is one's primary duty. Autonomy as effective deliberation requires more of health professionals. Respecting autonomy as effective deliberation requires a positive response in those instances in which there is a clear and discrete decision to be made. To ensure understanding, a health care provider may need to educate her patient, particularly if the choice involves complicated issues about which the patient has little previous understanding. Finally, the notion of autonomy as consistency raises perhaps the most far-reaching implications for health care professionals' behavior. The focus on consistency requires that the environment in which the elderly live be structured so as to allow individuals a chance to grow, to develop their own individual interests and goals, and to pursue the undertakings that they have chosen. This notion of autonomy requires health care professionals to take a much more active stance. As Agich comments:

> Respect for persons [autonomy] properly requires that we attend to their concrete individuality, to their effective and personal experiences; in short, we need to learn how to adapt to or at least to tolerate their habits and identifications. Nursing homes that respect autonomy must be open to the varied identifications that its elderly residents make and try to support them (Agich 1988:126).

The notion of autonomy as consistency, therefore, has particularly important implications for our study of autonomy in long-term care settings for the elderly. It requires us to understand that decisions do not occur independently of their context in a human self, and that assessing their autonomy requires focusing on that self, its history, current commitments, and foreseen future. Thus one critical aspect of understanding how the nursing home environment affects the autonomy of the elderly concerns how the elderly individual's persona is affected by the environment. Are the past activities, current identifications, and commitments and envisioned enterprises respected and encouraged or ignored and demeaned? It is the task of this research to try to describe the effects of a nursing home environment on autonomy in all of the above senses of the word.

NOTES

1. Much that the Nazi concentration camp physicians did had no scientific justification at all. However, the issue in the medical ethics debate is the legitimacy of

gathering information that might be scientifically valid but using procedures that violate standards of acceptability in the treatment of subjects.

2. Such desires are deeply encoded in our culture's commitment to individualistic values (Lidz 1983).

3. There is an obvious relationship between intention and understanding. At the least, to have intended to do something one must have a general idea about what it is that one intended to do. To use an extreme example, if someone signed what she thought was a consent to have a routine X-ray and it turned out that the consent was for major surgery, we would not think that she intended to have major surgery. Intentionality requires that a person have at least a minimal understanding about the act she plans to accomplish. She must, for example, understand that there is a connection between her behavior and certain consequences. However, this notion of understanding does not require the more complete understanding that is required for autonomy as effective deliberation.

4. Faden and Beauchamp use the term *controlled* rather than *involuntary*.

5. While we are not generally concerned here with whether or not a particular decision is voluntary, it is worth noting that deciding when an action is something that "I" wanted to do rather than something that "I" did only because of another's influence is often very difficult. Illegitimate influences often interfere with an individual's ability to evaluate her motivations. Christman (1988) recently offered one rule of thumb for distinguishing illegitimate from legitimate manipulation; an influence is illegitimate if a person would revise her action if she were aware of the factor's presence and its influence on her act. Take, for example, a patient who goes to occupational therapy only because the occupational therapist lied to her about what fun it was. If she had known the true facts about occupational therapy she would have never gone. This deception would therefore count as an illegitimate influence and we would conclude that the act was nonvoluntary and thus not autonomous. Thus, subliminal motivations, withholding of important information, and deception are generally considered illegitimate influences that decrease the voluntariness of an action.

6. It is more difficult to determine whether a physical infirmity also reduces the voluntariness of one's actions. What if it is a patient's Parkinson's Disease rather than her claustrophobia that prevents her from going into the elevator? These issues are beyond the scope of our analysis but are clearly important issues for the autonomy of the disabled elderly.

7. The ramification of this position is that health care professionals have an obligation to increase the patient's ability to effectively deliberate.

8. Whether what is required is optimizing rationality—the selection of that act that maximizes the chances of realizing the desired outcome—is a matter of some debate. Much of this literature seems to assume so but, as Simon has pointed out, such reasoning seems to be quite rarely done. More typical is what he calls "satisficing," which involves the search for a solution that is "good enough" for the purposes at hand.

9. We mean to use the term *enterprises* to refer to any project or endeavor in which an individual engages herself that involves a variety of different tasks over an extended period of time and requires at least some planning about how they are to be accomplished.

10. This formulation is clearer than the reality in that it presents a kind of pseudo-quantitative formulation of liberty issues. It is always possible to break down choices into an infinite number of smaller ones. Thus, a condemned prisoner on death row has the choice whether to walk to the electric chair quickly or slowly, to talk to his guards or not, to hang onto the bars and resist or cooperate, to smoke a cigar or not, etc. Even in this situation, it is possible to construct the situation so that the individual appears to have a limitless set of choices.

2

How Did We Get Here? A Brief History of the Nursing Home

Nursing homes are important institutions in our society. There are more than 19,000 of them in the United States and 2.3 million people reside in them at one time or another over a year's time. It is estimated that one person out of four will be in a nursing home at some time.

Although the remainder of this volume will consist of our findings about the institutional patterns and practices of a nursing home, it is appropriate to begin looking at the institution itself within its sociohistorical context. How did it come about that most of us think it reasonable that many elderly individuals should spend the last days, or even years, of their lives separated from their relatives, friends, and community, confined to a building with other elderly individuals? Moreover, why—within this setting—should they have many of the smallest details of their lives regulated by people whose training is in health care? Or, to put it more conventionally, how did our society come to accept as routine that nursing homes should be a major place to live for the elderly who cannot care for themselves without help?[1] Phrased that way the idea of the nursing home seems peculiar, a bizarre institution that functions as an arbitrary imposition on its residents. But nursing homes did not, like Athena, spring full-blown from the mind of Zeus. Our current medicalized, highly regulated approach represents the product of two centuries of continued effort to respond to the perceived needs of the elderly.

To understand the nature of our current system of long-term care for the elderly, we must examine the forces that contributed to the evolution of that system and provide the context in which it is maintained. This chapter will put institutional care for the elderly into historical perspective by exploring three major changes in the evolution of care for the elderly in American history. The first of these changes was the *rise of institutional care.* This happened within the context of the development of many other institutions for the management of a large variety of social problems (Rosenberg 1987). The second major change was *medicalization*, or the transfer of responsibility for such institutions from lay administrators who sought to produce personal character change to health care professionals who focused on the preservation of health. The final change was the growth of a complex, government-imposed *regulatory structure* that, in part, facilitated medicalization but has come increasingly to restrict the options of institutional authorities to provide different types of care for elderly residents. Each of these processes has had profound impacts on the autonomy of elderly individuals who need some sort of care or supervision. We will review these processes in their historical contexts.

The Colonial Period

Currently, we make numerous distinctions between the various types of people who need or demand different types of care and management. At this point in time, for example, no one would seriously contend that mental health treatment should be automatically imposed on the impoverished elderly or that orphans should be housed with alcoholics. However, while we see poverty, substance abuse, and parentless children as different problems, they are all social problems our society must manage. In contrast, in the eighteenth century the presence of deviant and dependent individuals—the poor, the sick, the disabled, and lawbreakers—was considered indigenous to society.

Colonial society clearly interpreted the presence of various needy and troublesome populations in a religious light. In a Puritan religious context in which the ultimate moral character of the individual was divinely fixed, these populations represented a divinely provided opportunity to fulfill one's charitable obligations. Consequently, the colonial approach to troublesome and dependent populations was not focused on personal change or reformation but on pragmatic and appropriate management. There were few attempts to treat the mentally ill, upgrade the poor, or rehabilitate the criminal. Rather, their management was attempted through direct, community-based actions. Specifically, financial or in-kind support was provided the ill and destitute within the community, while lawbreakers were dealt immediate punitive measures (such as whipping and execution). Notably, both the support structure and the beneficiaries of that support were local. Communities accepted collective responsibility for the care and management of their own dependent and difficult individuals.

It is also important to note that the help that was provided for the poor, (eg, food, clothing, housing, and small sums of money) was not systematic. Rather, problems were assessed more or less individually and solved with respect to convenience and frugality. Relatives, for example, were encouraged to assist, if not assume responsibility for, their needy kin. Likewise, individuals who required boarding were housed in the closest available homes, and the homeowners who volunteered to board the ill and indigent were rotated periodically. The elderly indigent and disabled were managed similarly to other indigent and disabled within this framework; what was done depended heavily on who their relatives were, whether or not their neighbors were willing to help, and other situation-specific factors.

Evaluation of the quality of care provided for dependent populations during this period is problematic because of the multitude of local variations, the scant number of specific records, and the diffuse nature of the care system. What we can say in its favor is that—although the amount of aid per person rarely extended beyond that needed to survive—the types of assistance provided the needy in the colonial period, unlike some later patterns of assistance, allowed the poor to remain in the community and thus maintain their social and familial roles.

Institutions for the care of dependents made their first appearance toward the latter part of the colonial period. The initial appearance of these facilities, however, did not reflect a change in the societal perspective on the problems of the poor or the elderly. Rather, as urban areas grew in size and complexity, providing assistance for dependents in these areas became increasingly difficult. Consequently, larger dwellings were established for the more efficient care of this population.

The first almshouses (or poor houses) were seen in cities like Boston, New York, and Philadelphia. These almshouses housed people so ill or disabled that they could not be maintained in the community, visitors who became too sick or incapacitated to travel, and an increasing number of dependents not manageable by less formal means. Again, however, these first almshouses reflected the problems of dealing with a greater number of cases on an individual basis rather than a noticeable shift in public attitude. Despite their size and urban location, many of these early almshouses were similar to private households in both social structure and appearance. Rather than building new structures, residential dwellings were often acquired and slightly modified to meet the needs of their occupants. Moreover, occupants were free to bring personal possessions into the almshouse and to dress in typical street clothes. The social structure of these almshouses was also quite similar to that of the traditional family; there were few staff or formal rules, and the more able-bodied residents participated in minor daily tasks.

Changes, however, began to be seen in the degree to which the personal characteristics of urban dependents were known to their caregivers. The colonial society that had relied exclusively on informal relief measures was a society of villages and small towns in which most people knew each other. Consequently, the personal characteristics of the needy were common knowledge. With the larger number of dependents cared for in the new urban almshouses, though, caregivers who had previous knowledge of those for whom they were providing care became more the exception than the rule.

The Rise of Institutions

During the last stages of the colonial period, assistance provided to the sick and indigent slowly began to be reformulated around a new focus on the causes of and cures for dependency. With it came a new preference for "indoor" (ie, institutional) rather than "outdoor" (ie, community-based) relief for the needy. While the focus on community responsibility remained a central feature of the late colonial approach to these problems, the practical means by which even the smallest communities dealt with dependents and criminals slowly began to shift from maintaining individuals in the community to a general policy of separating these individuals from the rest of society.

As this trend gathered momentum, almshouses, workhouses, insane and orphan asylums, and penitentiaries were built. While legislative bodies and philanthropists—slowly at first, but then with increasing enthusiasm—provided the funds necessary for construction, physicians and laypersons argued for their use.[2] Although these institutions developed first in large urban areas, they eventually became the standard in smaller urban and rural areas as well. In time, such settings became the first choice for managing social problems. With the increased specialization of function of these institutions (eg, creation of separate facilities for orphans, older indigents, lawbreakers, and the insane), the almshouse population became increasingly older. However, there was still little if any distinction made between the healthy but indigent elderly and the poor disabled elderly.

The Jacksonian Approach

Whereas the colonials believed dependency inherent to society and, therefore, focused on management rather than solutions, the Jacksonian era is characterized by the reconceptualization of deviancies as social problems (such as disability, poverty, and crime) that should not exist and that could be eliminated. Indeed, grounded on their optimistic view of the potentialities of the new nation, Jacksonians often seemed to see the very existence of such social problems as affronts to the national honor. Not surprisingly, as longstanding problems were redefined within a social framework, the approach to them in this period also became increasingly secular; the will of God was no longer accepted as a rationale for social differences.

Unfortunately, despite the increased use of institutions throughout this era, these problems continued to exist and, consequently, the focus of responsibility slowly began to shift away from society. Increasingly, dependents lost their positions as equal members of the community and began to be viewed as responsible for their own plight. Although some writers of the period made a distinction between the "worthy" and "unworthy" needy (eg, aged and orphans versus the able-bodied who would not work), their viewpoint did not dominate public policy. Rather, the possibility that corruption would spread became the primary consideration, and, consequently, citizens who were indigent, physically or mentally ill, or criminal were all seen as possible candidates for separation and rehabilitation.

The indigent or disabled elderly were similarly affected by this change in attitude. For them, the punitive nature of the almshouse was rationalized by the corresponding new health ideology which taught that poor moral habits were the cause of illness and dependency in old age. The prevailing opinion was that "anyone who lived a life of hard work, faith, and self-discipline could preserve health and independence to a ripe old age; the shiftless, faithless, and promiscuous, however, were doomed to premature death or a miserable old age" (Cole 1987:10).

Gradually, then, the colonial emphasis on compassion and the acceptance of responsibility for other community members disappeared. In its place, writers, theologians, and legislators focused on the causes of and cures for deviant behavior and dependency. In retrospect, the colonial approach was regarded as ineffective in that it passively encouraged new evils among a population by allowing the poor to avoid work and to indulge in vice. The new Jacksonian approach, on the other hand, was based on the belief that if the poor and unemployed had to rely on themselves, they would overcome their vices and become productive members of society.

Despite the emphasis on personal responsibility, however, most policymakers stopped short of assuming that all dependency was voluntary. Rather than being completely deprived of assistance, dependents were provided minimal aid in a dwelling separated from the community where it was believed that temptations to deviant behavior would be reduced and socially acceptable behavior encouraged. In particular, dependents were isolated from gambling, alcohol, and public handouts, and exposed to staff and "reformed" dependents as appropriate role models.

The new institutions of the Jacksonian era were quite different from their eighteenth century counterparts. Whereas the early colonial institutions for the poor and disabled were informal, largely unstructured systems that were modeled on large families, Jacksonian institutions were based on principles of order, discipline, and an exacting routine. Separation by age, health, and history was promoted in order to allow each institution to impose an appropriate kind of routine on its special population. For the able-bodied in workhouses this generally meant living in cells, taking meals at large tables in a collective dining area, wearing some items of clothing (such as striped caps) that clearly identified them as institution residents, and following a precise schedule for their daily routines.

Despite their intentions, Jacksonian institutions generally failed to achieve their rehabilitative goals; their primary success was in the effective separation of the ill, the indigent, and the criminal from the rest of society. Moreover, while this gap between goals and reality was considerable for all types of institutions, it appears to have been greatest in the almshouses where the original program goals were the least clear and public support minimal. In this setting, the principles of order, discipline, and an exacting routine were less likely to be implemented in a systematic fashion. Most almshouse or combination workhouse and almshouse residents were never systematically classified by type of disability, provided with regular work, or subjected to the strictly enforced discipline that many theorists thought would produce changes of character. Most often, both sexes were housed together, the insane and the ill were not separated, vagrants regularly came and went, no real work was provided for the able-bodied residents, and children remained uneducated.

Regardless, almshouses and workhouse and almshouse combinations of variable efficacy slowly spread from urban to rural areas. At best, cities maintained adequate facilities and smaller areas were able to at least feed and house the dependents. At worst, the needy lived in rundown buildings, with short rations and under conditions approaching abuse. The latter inspired periodic exposés of the quality of institutional care received by the residents of the almshouses. Rothman quotes the following excerpt from a New York State commission report:

> In an old dilapidated wooden building suitable only for an outbuilding . . . was found a demented old woman. She was in a state of turbulent dementia, scantily clad, barefoot, exceedingly filthy . . . the floor was wet and otherwise soiled with excrement, the odor from which was exceedingly offensive. In fact it smelled more like a privy vault than a place for the confinement of a human being (Rothman 1980: 30).

Despite the various institutional abuses highlighted in almshouses during the mid-nineteenth century, those disabled or indigent elderly not able to find support in the community were typically relocated to workhouses and almshouses. Although reformers of the period called for the correction of institutional abuses such as inadequate housing, poor food, filth, and general neglect, few advocated changes in the general system. Instead, the possibility of well-ordered, effective institutions combined with the influence of a growing institution lobby encouraged critics to advocate change from within.[3]

The persistence of institutions like the almshouse and the general shift from a focus on rehabilitation to custodial care is difficult to understand. Certainly one contributory factor was the public's conceptualization of institution residents as troublesome individuals with the capacity for corruption of others, individuals who were best separated from the rest of society (a view reinforced by the increased physical and emotional distance between the public and institutionalized individuals). Another possibility is that institution administrators truly succumbed to the misconception that, simply by holding people in custody, rehabilitation was taking place. For elderly individuals, there is substantial evidence that during this period of time there was a major deterioration of their prestige in society (Achenbaum 1978).

Once begun, the downward spiral from care and rehabilitation to custodianship continued unchecked. As institutions increasingly began to house chronic indigents and the severely disturbed, they developed increasingly negative reputations. Consequently, the less ill and disabled dependents in need of temporary help tried harder to avoid institutions. Administrators were forced, then, to focus their energies almost exclusively on managing the most difficult members of the population, thus undercutting services to the rest.

Regardless of causal interpretation, it is clear that society's techniques for managing the dependent elderly changed radically in the early nineteenth century. Public attitudes gradually shifted to endorse the goals of prevention, rehabilitation, and, eventually, simple custodianship. Despite the glaring inadequacies and poor reputations of existing facilities, the custodianship strategy of the later stages of the Jacksonian era remained effectively unchallenged until the twentieth century.

The Early Twentieth Century

The Progressive Era of the early twentieth century brought a new concern about the size and nature of the institutional population.[4] With the rise in immigration, this population was growing at a rapid pace, and concern over the financial ramifications of institutional populations soon became a topic for public debate. In addition, the presence of disabled elderly in almshouses (which were generally viewed as places of custody for the morally deficient) was beginning to arouse public discontent.

With the coming of the Great Depression, the almshouse—and public debate as to the appropriateness of institutionalization of the disabled or indigent elderly—came to play a major role in American political rhetoric. Of greatest relevance to our interests was the growing movement for a system of public pensions for the elderly grounded on the increasingly popular belief that it was immoral to relegate the elderly to almshouse life. Specifically, while financial dependency was still seen as a result of poor planning, there developed a general consensus "that chronic illness constituted a legitimate exception to the strictures of Puritan 'deservingness' " (Vladeck 1980:34).[5]

Social Security and the Advent of Proprietary Homes

Although there had been an increasing role for the medical and nursing professions in caring for the disabled elderly, the medical domination of institutions for the elderly did not occur until after the federal government became involved with homes for the elderly. That process began with the advent of the 1935 Social Security Act. The first governmental commitment to the elderly came in Title I of this act in the form of a public program referred to as Old Age Assistance (OAA), a temporary measure to meet the financial needs of the elderly until the Social Security Act was fully functional. This program provided partial federal matching of state-supported monthly payments of no more than $30 to recipients who met state-defined eligibility criteria.

One of the major principles of Social Security was that assistance recipients should be permitted to spend their benefits as they saw fit. Thus, the Social Security Act specifically disallowed the payment of OAA funds to institutionalized individuals.[6] The provision of cash awards to the community elderly, then, represented a reacceptance of dependents as community members with the right to choose the type of care they would receive.

Given the power of this new system, it is somewhat surprising that it had relatively little short-term impact on the almshouse system. Clearly, the most influential factor was the level of disability among almshouse residents. Specifically, many almshouse residents were simply unable to reside in the community, and it soon became clear that "pensions . . . were not a substitute for indoor relief, at least not for the elderly who were infirm as well as poor" (Vladeck 1980:37). The primary effect on the almshouse system of cash awards to the community elderly, then, was to increase the proportion of almshouse residents who were chronically ill or disabled by supplying the less disabled with the means to leave.

Although OAA payments did not provide for almshouse payments, OAA grants supported the growth of proprietary homes for the less impaired elderly. Despite the overwhelming emphasis on indoor relief during the Jacksonian period, the colonial practice of boarding dependents in private homes had never completely ceased. Now, spurred by the economic devastation of the depression and the availability of funding for community-based care, homeowners in need of income were encouraged to offer boarding to those indigent and disabled elderly who were manageable within a community setting. These entrepreneurial endeavors, referred to by some as "rest" or "convalescent" homes, typically involved "unemployed nurses [who]—either individually or in small, informal partnerships—would establish convalescent homes in their own home in hope of being able to pay the rent or meet the mortgage payment" (Vladeck 1980:37–38). Although the number of clients that could be accommodated in these home settings was limited, and the proportion of elderly initially serviced in this manner relatively small, the market for community care of the elderly, grounded on the OAA cash grants, soon flourished. Soon the size of the "homes" increased and the owners hired staff. Thus, what started out as an alternative to institutionalization became an alternative form of institution. Although Social Security was intended, in part, to provide the financial means for getting the impoverished elderly out of institutions, it developed into a new mechanism for funding institutions.

Almost from the start there was considerable discontent with the quality of care provided the elderly in convalescent homes. Documentation of abuses similar to those seen in the poorer almshouses reached public attention and was followed by public demand for the inspection of these proprietary homes. However, since there was a shortage of facilities, the calls for licensure were ignored, in the short run, in the hope that education and persuasion of "rest" and "convalescent" home operators would bring about the needed improvements.

The Emerging Medical Model

The growth of proprietary homes and the ongoing care provided by charitable organizations, both a result of OAA grant money, continued throughout the 1940s. Although there was little change in the financing of the care, some private homes began to make themselves more marketable by providing increasingly sophisticated medical care. Such a market-driven push to medicalization was not the only impetus for medicalization. Indeed, since perhaps the beginning of the century reformers had seen the professionalization of care as a means of upgrading the services provided to the elderly. Clearly the medical profession was the model that dominated these discussions. It is not surprising, then, that the liberal reform of the post-war era sought to encourage a medicalization of the care of the disabled elderly.

In the post-war era several legislative acts set the stage for our current health care policies. In 1946, Congress passed the Hill-Burton Act, which provided substantial funding for hospital construction. In 1950, amendments to the Social Security Act authorized payments to residents in public institutions, permitted direct payments to health care providers, and required states to begin licensing nursing homes. Of these amendments, the licensure requirement had the least immediate effect. While most states did develop regulations, "they varied enormously from one [state] to another, contained only the most minimal requirements, and were totally unenforced" (Vladek 1980:41). The second provision, permitting OAA payments to institution residents, reflected Congress's intent that counties and municipalities should convert what remained of the almshouse system into public facilities providing some level of health care. The provision allowing for direct payments to health care providers, though, had an immediate and significant impact on the growth of nursing homes. As it became clear that a profit could be made through the provision of care for the elderly, voluntary and, in particular, proprietary nursing homes, grew at a rapid rate.

In 1954 Congress amended the Hill-Burton Act to provide grants to nonprofit groups for the building of skilled facilities that met hospital-like building standards. Reflecting the desire of the Department of Health, Education, and Welfare to increase the quality of care offered in nursing facilities, nursing homes were included. Although public monies were limited to nonprofit organizations, this amendment consolidated some important changes in nursing home care. Specifically, the funding of these facilities with federal dollars put them under the Public Health Service, which administered the program. This transformed them, at least from an administrative perspective, into medical facilities.

Public nursing homes "were [now] redefined as the final stage of institutionalization for the chronically ill requiring long-term convalescence . . . ," and became part of "the prevailing ideology of 'progressive patient care,' in which patients were moved from one level of service intensity to another as their condition changed" (Vladeck 1980:43). Homes funded under the Hill-Burton amendment were subject to standards for design and construction, as well as staffing, that were heavily influenced by the hospital orientation of their designers. As a result, these new federally funded nursing care facilities functioned as extensions of hospitals by providing places of transfer for the elderly who, although not completely self-sufficient, did not require acute care. They also resembled hospitals in both structure and organization.

As the amount of public dollars needed to support the elderly in both public and private care facilities increased, so did public attention to how those dollars were spent. Despite the major impact of some provisions of the 1950 Social Security amendments, the standard-setting portion of the amendment was of little practical consequence since it specified no minimum standards or procedures, and there was no mechanism for assuring state enforcement. The development of effective licensing and other regulation remained for a later era in the history of nursing homes.

The 1960s opened with the passing of the Kerr-Mills Act, which replaced OAA with a program referred to as Medical Assistance for the Aged (MAA). Kerr-Mills allowed states to set their own criteria for determining "medical indigency" and removed the ceiling on federal matching. This act had a substantial impact on the continued growth of nursing homes. By 1965 more than half of all nursing home residents were beneficiaries of Kerr-Mills payments for nursing home services and close to one-third of the program monies (roughly $449 million) was being paid for their care.

Lyndon Johnson's landslide victory in 1964 provided the votes to pass the Medicare Act (Title XVIII of the Social Security Act) the next year. While this Act's major impact was to provide entitlement funding for medical care for the elderly, its impact on nursing homes was through its allocation of funding for individuals over 65 years old who required up to 100 days of convalescence in what were referred to as "extended care facilities," or ECFs. This program also specified that "facilities eligible to be reimbursed for extended care [be limited] to those either formally affiliated, or maintaining a written 'transfer agreement' for patients and their records, with a general hospital" (Vladeck 1980:241). By developing the "extended care facility" concept, creators of this program attempted to control costs by distinguishing reimbursable skilled care from that customarily provided in proprietary and voluntary nursing facilities. The result was to further encourage the development of hospital-like services in an effort to qualify for reimbursement under this new program. Once again, in an effort to upgrade the care provided to the disabled elderly, Congress had further medicalized their care.

Also included in the Social Security amendment of 1965 was an appendage referred to as Medicaid, a program designed to provide health care benefits to any individual who either received federal welfare payments or met the state-defined "medical indigency" criteria. Among the five basic mandated services was "skilled nursing homes." Regulations specified that the regulation of skilled nursing homes under Medicaid was to be the same as that for an extended-care facility under Medicare.

The Growth of Regulation

One immediate effect of these programs was a tremendous increase in the amount of public monies available for elderly health care. Perhaps more important, though, were the major new regulations concerning the type of facilities to be reimbursed as nursing homes under this new program. They were extensive and in many ways mimicked hospital regulations.

Not surprisingly, few nursing homes could meet these new standards. As this became apparent (only slightly over ten percent of the first 6000 applicant facilities were completely eligible), a compromise was reached; the Bureau of Health Insurance created a new Medicare facility designation, "substantial compliance," which was designed to allow facility participation for a period of time during which those facilities would work to achieve complete compliance. Later amendments (1967) created the "intermediate-care facility," for those individuals "who needed medical services less intensive than those provided by skilled nursing homes but more intensive than nothing . . ." (Vladeck 1980:63). Intermediate care was intended to provide long-term custodial care for those who could not function without it. The less stringent standards contained in this legislation allowed facilities unable to meet even substantial compliance eligibility to qualify for Medicaid vendor payments.

Despite the intended use of substantial compliance as an interim measure, there is little evidence that homes certified as being in substantial compliance improved very much. Intermediate care facility certification was not much better. While some states arbitrarily reclassified skilled patients and facilities as intermediate, other states used this new designation to gain certification for facilities unable to meet even the most basic fire and safety standards.

In hindsight, it appears clear that the Johnson administration had little idea as to where nursing homes should fit into their health care package. Cognizant that care of the chronically ill elderly was frequently more custodial than curative, Medicare strategists were afraid the nursing home industry would become a bottomless financial pit. However, under the belief that utilizing nursing homes instead of hospitals to care for patients in the last stages of recuperation or illness would provide economic benefits, limited nursing home coverage was included in both the Medicare and Medicaid legislation.

The initiation of the Medicare and Medicaid programs changed the nature of nursing homes forever. These programs provided seemingly unlimited federal and matching federal funds for facilities able to provide hospital-like services in a hospital-like atmosphere. As a result, the nursing home industry got a financial shot in the arm as a reward for becoming more embedded in the medical model. The cost of this increase in funding, however, was a maze of new regulations.

The next two decades were filled with legislative amendments, each designed to provide greater control over what was quickly becoming a fiscal and quality-control disaster. A congressional hearing chaired by Senator Howard Moss provided repeated examples of a wide variety of abuses leading to greater regulatory efforts. For our interests, however, only one attempt at modification prior to our study was significant. In 1974, the Nursing Home Affairs study looked at the structure and management of 288 of the newly designated "skilled nursing facilities," and concluded that regulation surveys assessed only the ability to deliver, rather than the actual delivery of services, by facilities, and that there was considerable variation in the degree to which these facilities complied with federal regulations. Under the direction of the Carter administration, the Office of Long-term Care initiated a revision of the skilled nursing facility standards for care, focusing on the medical nature of the regulations, the lack of emphasis on outcome measures, and the overwhelming paperwork related to these standards. In general, the new rules resulted in shifting the focus away from the paper-documented ability of facilities to provide particular services and toward an evaluation of patients and the care that they were actually receiving.

These regulations were widely thought of as a progressive step toward improving the lives of people residing in nursing homes. However, they faced intense resistance from the nursing home lobby, which was concerned about the cost of these changes. Most of the proposed regulations remained unpassed until the very end of the Carter administration. The Reagan administration immediately rescinded the new regulations in favor of their own regulatory reform effort, one which proved so unacceptable to legislators, nursing home owners, and consumer groups that it was dropped. Later efforts to amend the standards also met considerable resistance.

The Regulatory Criteria at the Time of This Study

While there have been some additional changes since our study (to be discussed below), at the time of the field work, government regulation of nursing homes consisted of a complicated process by which states granted nursing homes the right to operate. In spite of subsequent changes, the fundamental features of the regulatory environment are still in place. We will limit our attention here to the regulations governing the operation of nursing homes and the methods by which they are used to determine facility compliance.

Standards

There were, at the time of the study, two different sets of federal operational criteria for the certification of nursing homes. The first set of criteria related to SNFs (skilled nursing facilities) and spanned ninety standards of care ranging from physical environment to social services. A second set of regulations for ICFs (intermediate care facilities) detailed roughly half as many care standards across a variety of nursing facility service categories. These two sets of regulations, however, were (and still remain) quite similar in their level of complexity and overwhelming attention to detail.[7]

While both skilled and intermediate standards emphasize quality medical care, physical safety, and sanitation measures in great detail (eg, the number and types of staff required for each shift, appropriate food-handling techniques, and required fire and safety measures), they also address, to a lesser degree, select quality-of-life issues (such as required patient-resident activities and social services programs, the conditions under which physical and chemical restraints may be used, and the right of patients to privacy and to knowledge of treatment and discharge plans). The majority of both SNF and ICF standards, however, are focused on health and safety measures and, within those areas, on the ability of facilities to follow specific procedures in providing particular services. Recent changes in the regulations focused on aide training and patient's rights, as we will discuss below, but have not fundamentally changed this pattern.

Various evaluations of the nursing home regulatory system have led to the conclusion that, although nursing home regulations are somewhat successful in standardizing the capability of facilities to provide particular services, they tend to overemphasize procedures and the ability to provide services while underemphasizing the quality of care actually provided (Abdellah 1978, Anderson & Stone 1969). In other words, the current standards do not ensure either adequate provision of services or quality of life for nursing home patients.

Certification

The certification of nursing homes is a joint effort of the federal and state governments. In general, the survey process by which inspections are effected is designed to "identify and measure performance deficiencies that result in poor-quality care and should provide documentation of the deficiencies that will support the government's case in contested enforcement actions" (Vladeck 1980:104). While the standards are set by both federal and state governments, the inspection of homes for adherence to standards is the responsibility of the individual states. Certification for Medicaid participation is done directly by state agencies, while Medicare-only or mixed certification is effected by the Health Care Finance Agency (HCFA) regional offices on the basis of state recommendations. In either case, however, the federal government also has the authority to inspect and decertify substandard facilities.

Much criticism has been aimed at this certification process. First, despite their detail, many of the regulations use vague terms that necessitate interpretation on the part of nursing home inspectors, a situation further complicated by considerable variance in their training and experience (Institute of Medicine 1986). The result is inconsistency in the application of standards across facilities. In addition, measurement of compliance is dichotomous (a facility is either in compliance or not in compliance), and is made without reference to case mix within and across facilities. Further, the survey process focuses on paper compliance rather than observation and patient interviews. While these shortcomings may hinder medical and safety regulation, their impact is necessarily greater on the more difficult to measure quality-of-life issues, to say nothing of even vaguer concepts like patient autonomy. Despite the existence of standards to regulate some aspects of quality of life within nursing homes, then, only the most quantitative (and, perhaps, least meaningful) of these standards (eg, minimum number of square feet per patient room) can be accurately and consistently evaluated.

Both the federal government and individual states have a variety of sanctions for the enforcement of regulations. Courses of action available to the federal government include required plans of correction and a variety of more forceful sanctions. State sanctions vary considerably and range from the withholding of payments and suspension of admissions to license revocation and criminal penalties. Federal actions, in particular, are usually directed at improving facility performance rather than merely requiring strict adherence to regulatory standards.[8]

In general, the current system of nursing home regulation only marginally achieves its primary objective—to provide high-quality medical care in a safe, clean environment. The regulations, while clearly focused on medical care and safety issues, are complex, vague, and unwieldy. The inspection process is performed by persons varying considerably in expertise and focuses on minimal paper compliance with objectively defined standards. Further, the compliance process is relatively ineffective, allowing marginal homes to continue in operation and, in effect, permitting poor-quality care (Abdellah 1978, Rauchlin 1980).

From the point of view of promoting autonomy in the nursing home, at the time of our study, the regulations barely touched on the important issues. Indeed, these regulations promoted various procedural rigidities that strongly encouraged the staff to restrict patients' freedom.

In an effort to remedy these and other problems, as part of the Omnibus Budget Reconciliation Act (OBRA) of 1987, Congress mandated a variety of new regulations including provisions requiring that aides receive some basic types of training, primarily focused on safety and health but including training in residents' rights. More importantly for our purposes, they provided some specific rights for residents of nursing facilities. We will discuss this part of the OBRA regulations after describing our findings because our comments should be understood in light of the findings.

Conclusion

This chapter has traced the development of long-term care for the disabled elderly from the informal procedures of the small towns of the colonial period to the present highly regulated and medicalized institutions. We have seen the development of three fundamental changes that substantially affect the autonomy of the disabled elderly in long-term care. The first of these was the rise of institutions—first public almshouses, then convalescent homes, and finally modern nursing homes. The transition to the nursing home reflected the second change, the pervasive medicalization of care that turned these institutions into hospital-like facilities. Finally, we have seen the growth of governmental attempts to regulate these institutions in the interests of the health and safety of their patients. The rest of this book will focus on the impact of these institutions on the autonomy of the elderly individuals who live in them.

NOTES

1. Of course, nursing homes are not the exclusive residence of the elderly. Many young and middle-aged disabled persons reside in these care settings. Our interest, however, is in the elderly receiving long-term care in nursing facilities.

2. Several theories have been proposed to explain this change in approach from community management to institutionalization. Rothman (1971), however, convincingly argues that the trend toward institutionalization was first and foremost an attempt to deal with problems (such as crime, poverty, and severe illness) conceptualized for the first time as social in nature. He contends that institutions were seen as possessing both preventive and restorative functions; they could "rehabilitate" deviants by separating them from the rest of society (which was assumed to be the source of their problems) and by providing them with examples of appropriate behavior.

3. The absence of a real demand for improved institutional conditions might also have reflected the fact that such facilities were generally the homes for the immigrant poor rather than the wealthy or the Yankees who dominated the political and intellectual life of the era. The wealthy established private homes for the indigent and disabled aged who had the proper social background (Cole 1987).

4. In what follows we have leaned very heavily on Vladeck's fine study, *Unloving Care: The Nursing Home Tragedy*, New York: Basic Books, 1980. We have not cited our dependence on his work for routine background information but only for quotations and opinion.

5. It should be noted that public debate over the most appropriate housing for the dependent elderly obscured the fact that relatively few elderly people actually lived in almshouses. In fact, approximately the same number of dependent elderly were cared for in private homes supported by various charities as resided in almshouses (Vladeck 1980). However, because the cost of care in these private facilities was not borne by the public, they did not merit the same public interest and scrutiny as those supported by public monies. Thus, the development and utilization of these private care facilities went relatively unnoticed and did not have the impact on the regulatory decision-making that public facilities had.

6. This, in part, reflected increasing public discontent with the almshouse system, which had been fanned by the Townsend Movement advocates for a universal old-age pension system.

7. The SNF "conditions of participation" standards for care are distributed across the following areas: state licensure, administrative body, medical direction, physician and nursing care, rehabilitation, transfer, physical environment, utilization review, infection control and disaster preparedness, the recording of medical information, and dietary, pharmacy, laboratory or testing, dental, recreational, and social services. The forty-six ICF regulations are grouped into the following seven categories: administrative methods and procedures, safety standards, environmental and sanitation standards, meal service, medications, health services, and "other" services.

8. Aspects of the process component also contribute to the general effectiveness

of compliance proceedings. (1) The entire process is partially compromised by the ability of some nursing homes to predict (or gain access to) the times of upcoming inspections and bring their performance temporarily into compliance. (2) The intensity of nursing home inspections is relatively equal across homes, including those with poor compliance histories. (3) Since errors of commission (citations) are generally riskier than errors of omission (overlooking a violation), it is likely that surveyors focus on more visible violations at the expense of less visible, more interpretative (and more likely related to quality-of-life) violations (Diver, 1980). (4) Nursing homes are given an extension during which they can improve their performance. Noncompliant homes are typically given additional compliance time past the point at which formal sanctions could be legally imposed.

3

The Research Setting and Strategies

We undertook this research in order to describe how different institutional structures either enhance or erode autonomy in long-term care settings. Unlike the acute care settings on which the medical ethics literature has focused, long-term care is an all-encompassing phenomenon that affects all aspects of patients' lives and, therefore, their autonomy. Although it might have been easier for us to concentrate on the major decisions regarding care and treatment (ie, admission, discharge, and termination of life supports), these are infrequent decisions that have little to do with the day-to-day lives of those who live in long-term care settings.[1] Consequently, we chose to focus our attention on the routine interactions between staff and patients or residents that form the core of the latter's daily existence. We will discuss various aspects of these interactions throughout the remainder of this book. First, however, it is helpful to describe the context in which our data was collected and analyzed.

The Research Setting

Physical Layout

This research was done at a relatively large geriatric facility owned by a nonprofit health system. Originally a small hospital, this facility had been remodeled and expanded to encompass two skilled, one intermediate, and one mixed skilled and intermediate patient units, and a three-unit independent living area. Occupant capacity was over 150, and there was generally a waiting list for admission to the patient units. The combined intermediate and skilled patient care units contained over 100 beds, roughly two-thirds for skilled and one-third for intermediate care.

The independent living area, commonly referred to as the "residence," had over 30 beds and was spread out over three different floors of the building. This area was, however, in a separate wing completely separated from the patient units. Residents, their visitors, and the residential staff used a private elevator. Not surprisingly, interactions between residents and patients were limited to the larger communal areas such as the dining hall and activity rooms. However, there was a clear reluctance on the part of residents to interact with patients even in the communal settings. For example, residents frequently complained about taking meals in the same area with patients. The facility responded to these complaints by planning a wall to separate the portion of the dining hall in which residents ate from that used by patients.

Patients and Residents

We observed two patient units (one intermediate, one mixed skilled and intermediate) housing about 30 patients each at any one time. In the residence, two of the three floors, housing about 30 residents, were occupied during our project.[2] We collected data on a total of 66 patients and on all 30 residents.

Despite their respective units, the patients and residents were quite similar in many ways. The mean age of both groups was almost identical (patient mean = 83.8; resident mean = 83.6). Both groups were predominantly white (patients = 95%; residents = 100%) and, as expected for this age group (Uhlenberg, 1987), there was a preponderance of females (female patients = 85%; female residents = 90%). Nearly the same percentage of each group had at least one family member residing within convenient driving distance of the facility (patients = 38%; residents = 40%).

There were, however, some differences between patient and resident groups with regard to other sociodemographic variables. The patient group was predominantly Protestant (49%), while a plurality of the residents was Catholic (43%). Slightly more patients than residents were widowed (patients = 61%; residents = 50%), while half of the residents (as opposed to roughly one-third of the patient group) resided in their own homes prior to admission to this facility.

There were also differences in the comparative length of stay in the facility. The majority of patients in both skilled and intermediate care had lived at the nursing home more than three years (mean length of patient stay = 4.37 years; standard deviation (s.d.) = 4.33).[3] Most residents, on the other hand, had lived in this facility for less than one year (83%). Further, although patients in skilled and intermediate care and residents had roughly the same number of diagnoses (skilled = 3.1; intermediate = 3.2; residents = 3.2), the medical reasons underlying their need for care varied considerably.[4]

As we will discuss below, nurses and aides reliably rated both patients and residents on five dimensions: ability to make rational decisions, mobility, assertiveness, ability to manage activities of daily living, and ability to live independently. Staff rated most patients as being impaired across these dimensions, the exception being patients' ability to manage activities of daily living (eg, eating, dressing, oral hygiene, etc.). However, it is important to remember that the cut-off point is ultimately arbitrary. In general residents were rated as less impaired on these criteria, reflecting in part the different admission criteria. However, as will be discussed later, there are substantial overlaps on all distributions.

As we have noted, the residents looked very much like the patients in many respects. In theory, residents were supposed to be continent, mobile, and cognitively able to manage their own affairs. However, because of the recent expansion of the independent living area and the need to fill the beds, the only criterion firmly enforced was that of physical mobility. All residents were required to undergo an evaluation to assure staff that they could meet this criterion prior to admission. The staff to resident ratio of 1:15 precluded admitting individuals whose ability to ambulate was compromised. Although infrequent post-admission exceptions were made (eg, the dietary service would send food up to a resident in bed with the flu), residents whose mobility was compromised for more than a few days were transferred.

Staff

Staff were divided in two slightly overlapping hierarchies: one predominantly concerned with running the facility (management hierarchy) and the other focused on direct patient and resident care (caregiving hierarchy).

Dimension	*Percent Patients Impaired*	*Percent Residents Impaired*
Rational decision-making	82	30
Mobility	51	20
Assertiveness	65	35
Activities of daily living	37	20
Independent living	89	83

Administrators sat at the highest levels of the management hierarchy. They were largely uninvolved in the day-to-day care decisions, although their decisions had a significant impact on routine care. Below the administrators were a variety of quasi-professionals, some whom were solely responsible to administration (eg, admissions coordinator, patient accounts representatives), while others were involved in both administrative decisions and direct patient care (eg, nursing supervisors and social services). The repetitive tasks necessary to run the facility were the responsibility of lower-level management hierarchy employees, grouped into departments on the basis of function (eg, maintenance, dietary, and housekeeping). While not directly involved in either decision-making or patient care, these staff nonetheless interacted with many patients and residents during the performance of their tasks.

Physicians occupied the highest status within the caregiving hierarchy; however, they were rarely present at the facility and typically gave orders over the phone at the request or suggestion of staff or families. Thus, most caregiving was provided by the nurses and aides. Several specialized staff, such as the clinical specialist, nursing supervisors, and social worker, held positions of authority just below that of the physicians. These staff fit into both the caregiving and management hierarchies and were responsible to patients, their families, and the administration. The decisions of specialized staff regarding admissions, discharges, and available staffing affected not only the population of the facility, but the types and length of specific treatments provided to patients.

While these specialized staff contributed to the running of the facility, they also had specialized care or treatment responsibilities. Nursing supervisors directed the line staff who provided the routine unit care. The clinical specialist supervised treatment issues at this and two other health system facilities, and played an active role in continuing staff education. The social worker managed placements, while the physical and occupational therapists provided their respective specialized services. All of these individuals were seen as sitting at roughly the same level in the system. They met together regularly and, unlike the direct care staff, had assigned office spaces away from the patient care areas. While they had considerable power in the system, they, like physicians, were not responsible for direct patient care on a daily basis. As a group we will refer to them as upper staff.

The direct care staff on patient units were the registered and practical nurses, and personal care aides. The charge nurses for the skilled and intermediate units, who supervised the other nurses and aides working on those units, were generally RNs during the day and evening and LPNs at night. On the intermediate unit, however, all charge nurses were LPNs. Charge nurses were accountable to the nursing supervisors, but were not directly supervised by any other upper level staff. These staff spent any time they had that was not involved in patient care in small lounges located on the patient units.

While there was always a charge nurse (either RN or LPN) on each unit regardless of the time of day, the presence of a second nurse and the number of personal care aides varied according to the shift. In general, a second nurse (usually an LPN) and four personal care aides assisted the charge nurse on both the skilled and intermediate units during the 7 AM to 3 PM shift. From 3 to 11 p.m. each of the two units are staffed with one nurse and three to four personal care aides, while the 11 PM to 7 AM staffing consisted of one nurse (LPN on both units) and two aides.

It should be noted that nurses' training differs from that of aides and monitors in both length and nature. Despite some emphasis on routine aspects of care, the training of both LPNs and RNs emphasizes clinical skills and prepares nurses for technical tasks, such as inserting nasogastric tubes and IV administration. Their training (full-time study through an accredited program lasting from one to four years) focused on the management and treatment of acute medical conditions. For personal care aides, on the other hand, formal training was rare.[5] Prior training in the field was usually via prior employment rather than schooling. Instead of emphasizing technical medical skills, the aides' job description assumed aides would spend most of their time assisting patients with activities of daily living such as bathing, dressing, and eating.

Despite differences in training and job descriptions, the duties of nurses and aides (particularly on the intermediate unit) were quite similar. Their responsibilities differed primarily in that nurses administered medications and had more extensive charting responsibilities. Although nurses were more likely to use their clinical skills with patients in the skilled care units, even within that setting the duties of nurses and aides overlapped considerably. Overall, then, the work afforded both nurses and aides on the mixed skilled and intermediate and the intermediate units was quite routine.

The residential unit care hierarchy was somewhat simpler. Because admissions were arranged directly through administration, the admissions coordinator was not involved with this part of the facility. Supervision of the residential direct care staff (monitors) from 7 AM to 11 PM was handled by one of two residential nursing supervisors (both LPNs) who, in turn, were supervised by the clinical specialist. On the night shift supervision of the residential care staff was assumed by the night nursing supervisor for the patient units.

The lowest members of the care hierarchy in the residential setting are referred to as monitors. Despite their similarity in status to personal care aides, monitors differed substantially from aides in their training, prior work experiences, and duties. Resident monitors, for the most part, had no formal training. Although some had experience working in health service positions (eg, home companion, assisting the mentally retarded in group homes), most monitors were housewives looking for additional income. In the words of one upper staff member, the monitors were just "people off the street." They learned the needed skills on the job by spending shifts with the nurses who supervised residential care and with other monitors. Although they occasionally assisted residents in various activities of daily living (ADLs), most of their time was spent accompanying residents to the dining hall and facility activities, making medical appointments, and arranging transportation for off-grounds activities. Monitors provided much less hands-on assistance with ADLs than the aides. Both upper staff and monitors refered to the position as that of "facilitator," as most of the monitors' time and effort was spent on helping residents interact with the outside world.

Finally, several points may be compared between patient and resident line staff. Nurses (LPNs and RNs) and aides on the patient units were similar in age (the average age was in the mid-forties) and, without exception, female. They were somewhat less similar relative to length of employment (mean = 7 years for nurses, 10 years for aides), and strikingly different in race, ie, 64% of the nurses were white, while 63% of the aides were black. While resident monitors were similar to nurses and aides in both age (mean age = 43) and gender (all female), they were more evenly divided relative to race (55% black, 45% white).

Research Strategy—The Use of Participant Observational Techniques

This project required an intensive study of the relationships between patients or residents, families, and the staff in two distinctly different institutional settings, ie, patient (both skilled and intermediate) and residential units. Our data collection technique, a type of augmented ethnography, lent itself well to these goals. We relied primarily on nearly verbatim transcriptions of interpersonal interactions, interpreted within their context and supplemented with observational, interview, and artifactual data. This provided us with the raw material to describe the daily routine of these settings.

In order to gather sufficient data on the issues we introduced in Chapter 1, however, it was necessary to make some modifications in traditional ethnographic methods. First, rather than attemptng to describe completely the entire institutional setting, we focused on gathering information that shed light on patient autonomy. This information included descriptions of patient, staff, and family role definitions, the value complexes surrounding those roles, and the normative structures of the institution that regulated patients' activities. Further, to adequately describe how the institutional structure affected autonomy, we spent a large amount of time observing routine staff-patient-family interactions. Such observations often produced a vivid picture of the patients' day-to-day lives. Consider the following example taken from observation of the day room on one unit.

> Observation: *Mrs. Martine (an elderly, white woman dressed in a nightgown and robe) is . . . sitting [in her wheelchair] in the hallway. She continues to struggle with her afghan. Kathleen, the charge nurse, is sitting in a nearby room talking to a patient. The door is halfway closed. George Anderson (an anemic-looking white man in his late eighties with visible symptoms of Parkinson's disease) and wife Evelyn (who is visiting) are sitting in the television lounge. . . . Mrs. Friedman (an elderly, aphasic Jewish woman) is sitting in the wheelchair by the elevator. She is crying silently with her mouth open. As I pass, she tries to grab me. Mrs. Anderson moves her husband to a different area of the lounge and sits down in a chair near him. Meanwhile, Ruth (an aide) empties the garbage bag in the lounge. She brings the trash back down the hallway.*
>
> MRS. ZELKAN (a severely demented patient who is sitting in the middle of the day room): Nurse!
>
> Observation: *There is no response.*
>
> MRS. ZELKAN: Nurse! (louder)
>
> KERRY (an aide): What? (yelling down the hallway)
>
> MRS. ZELKAN: Is this on the wrong side?
>
> Observation: *Kerry walks up the hallway to Mrs. Zelkan. She is struggling with her sweater. It appears to be on inside out.*
>
> KERRY: I think so. (laughing)
>
> MRS. ZELKAN: I have another one.
>
> KERRY: I'll take care of it.
>
> Observation: *Kerry walks away. [I move to the lounge].*
>
> MRS. KRAMER (a tall, very thin patient in her nineties): Oh, oh, oh, oh, oh, oh (etc.) (smacking her lips)
>
> Observation: *Mrs. Kramer is dressed in purple knee socks and a pink*

> *robe and is wearing a pink hair ribbon. As she sings, she grabs my hand.*
> MRS. ZELKAN: Nurse! Come here!
> Observation: Kathleen rolls a cart up the hallway and into the lounge . . . . She is pouring grape juice and dispensing medications.
> MRS. KRAMER: Oh, oh, oh, oh, god. (then begins humming)
> MRS. ZELKAN: Nurse! Please!
> MRS. KRAMER: Hum, hum, hum (etc.)
> MRS. ZELKAN: Nurse! Come here! Please come here!
> Observation: *Kathleen continues to administer medications . . . .*
> MRS. KRAMER: Hmm, hmm, oh, oh. (etc.) (rocking from side to side)
> MRS. ZELKAN: Nurse! Please come here! Nurse! Come here!
> Observation: *Mrs. Kramer continues to hum. . . . Mr. Anderson is drooling a lot. He's tied in a wheelchair and is wearing a rubber bib. He slowly rolls himself forward and backwards. His wife sits in a chair and watches.*
> MRS. ZELKAN: Nurse! Please come here! Please!
> TV: "I'm doing the best that I can for my family with this [fabric] softener."
> MRS. ZELKAN: Nurse! Nurse!
> MRS. KRAMER: Hm, hm, hm, oh, oh, oh . . .
> Observation: *Kathleen rolls the cart down the hallway. It appears that she's finished administering meds. . . . There are 11 people in the television lounge. Mrs. Kramer is singing, Mrs. Zelkan is yelling, and Mr. Anderson is drooling. The others, with the exception of visitors, appear to be in various stages of stupor. . . .*

As the result of this observation technique, much of our data consists of verbatim interactions (such as that shown above) described within broader behavioral observations. A key advantage of this approach is the availability of considerable information on the **nature** of the context in which specific interactions are embedded.

To understand the ways in which decisions about care and treatment were made, observers attended discharge and planning meetings, and care conferences. These meetings were held at regular intervals to address the continued treatment and disposition of patients. Weekly discharge and planning meetings were attended by the facility director, the clinical specialist, the day shift nursing supervisor, the admissions coordinator, the social worker, and the occupational and physical therapists. Several patient cases were generally presented at each hour-long meeting. Typically the nursing supervisor or clinical specialist presented a synopsis of each patient's medical condition and past illnesses, followed by an open discussion of the patient's response to treatment, amount of remaining insurance coverage (or other method of payment), and prognosis. Below is an excerpt from one such meeting.

> UPPER STAFF–01:[6] OK, this is Mrs. Owen. She is 54, and this is her second admission here. She was home just one day, fell, and fractured her hip. She also has multiple other problems including a skin disease, congestive heart failure, chronic obstructive pulmonary disease, a deep venous thrombosis, and so on.
> US–05: What is her skin disease?
> US–01: Mycoses fungoides . . . . She came in about two weeks ago. We are probably going to send her home if her fracture heals well enough. Will we have enough insurance or will there be problems?
> US–06: She is insured by [private insurance] and has approximately 100 days . . . .
> US–07: She is really gun shy in [physical] therapy. She fell in rehab before.
> US–02: Do you see her as being able to live independently in a wheelchair? Would she have problems?
> US–07: That depends on how she does. She just doesn't have any endurance.
> US–06: Does she have family?
> US–02: Yes, they are really good. Her husband was with her when she fell. She might not be so afraid if she was in a wheelchair and independent . . . .
> US–05: She is independent of ADLs (activities of daily living). If you decide she is wheelchair independent, we will need to go in the home and get things arranged.
> US–07: I think the amount of time it will take . . . the hospital time will probably run out before we have her up and walking . . . .

We also attended the weekly care conferences on each of the patient units. These conferences were typically chaired by either the social worker or clinical specialist, and attended by the day shift charge nurse and a variable number of personal care aides. The family members of patients to be discussed were invited but generally did not attend. The format was less formal and less medically oriented than the discharge and planning meetings. Case histories were rarely presented, and the primary focus was on the ability of patients to manage activities of daily living and on specific post-discharge care arrangements. These conferences gave us insight into how health professionals conceptualized patients and how such beliefs affected decisions about the care of patients.

We also employed other modifications of traditional ethnography. Rather than relying on the observers' ability to remember key aspects of observed interactions, the observers recorded conversations using a form of speedwriting (Grossman 1976). This method results in nearly verbatim transcripts and has been shown in previous studies to have a high degree of interobserver reliability (Lidz et al 1983, 1984). Speedwriting was used primarily in communal areas where a variety of individuals were interacting and the observers were able to remain relatively unobtrusive, or in formal meetings in which note-taking fit in with the activity of others. In situations where note-taking was likely to have more of an effect, however, we simply watched and listened so as to preserve rapport and minimize our effect on the behavior of those individuals under observation. Fortunately, as time passed, staff and patients became accustomed to our presence, and it became possible to record conversation in almost every type of interaction.

Finally, since we worked as a team, we were forced to make other modifications in traditional ethnographic methods. For example, we routinely reviewed notes together and discussed observations and analyses by various members of the project. We also did much of our analysis using a computer program designed to organize and access field notes. We will discuss data analysis in more detail later in this chapter.

Nonethnographic Data Collection

Our intention was to observe both inpatient units and in the independent (residential) living area. While we gathered approximately one hundred hours of observation spanning a roughly equal distribution of days, nights, and weekends in both of the patient settings, the design of the independent living area limited our use of participant observation. There was almost nothing to observe unobtrusively in the residential communal areas because of the physical structure of this setting (eg, one of the three independent living areas had no communal area) and the considerable amount of time residents spent in their rooms and outside the facility.

While we sought to avoid intrusive and obtrusive data collection procedures, we supplemented our approximately fifty hours of observation of the interactions of residents in larger communal areas (eg, dining hall, activity rooms) with many resident interviews and resident staff interviews. These interviews were tape recorded, thus allowing the observers to play a more active role in suggesting topics and asking specific questions. Though not highly structured, all interviews followed a similar format; those being interviewed were encouraged to talk about their background and what they did before becoming associated with the facility, their experiences within the setting, characterizations of those within the facility with whom they interacted, and their concerns for the future. Overall, we interviewed nine upper staff, twelve line staff (nurses and aides), three patients and six residents. Some individuals (in particular, upper staff) were interviewed numerous times.

Despite the interviews we encountered problems in comparing the data collected from the independent living area with that gathered on the two patient units. Specifically, while all the line and supervisory independent living staff consented to interviews, we had relatively little observational data by which to examine typical resident-resident and resident-staff interactions.

Moreover, most of the cognitively unimpaired residents refused project participation. As a result, while there is considerable consistency across residential staff interviews, we had little noninterview data with which to validate staff's portrayal of life in this setting. Throughout the analyses we remained aware that much of our information on the residential area was from the staff perspective, and kept this in mind when analyzing the independent living data.

In addition to interviews, we collected two other types of data—assessment rating scales and medical and demographic information. In order to gather systematic evidence on the general staff views of patients' capabilities and situations, we asked nurses and aides on each unit to complete identical, six-item, seven-point Likert scales for each patient or resident who participated in this study. This scale was constructed specifically for this study and allowed staff to rate each patient or resident on six dimensions:

1. Ability to make rational decisions independently.
2. Walking without aid or restriction.
3. Assertiveness about making decisions.
4. Ability to manage ADLs independently.
5. Familial involvement in care decisions.
6. Likelihood of living independently in the near future.

The scale was completed by both the unit charge nurse and a primary care aide. Interclass correlations revealed a moderately high degree of concordance ($\geq .7$) between these two ratings across all scale items except item 5, which we dropped from the analysis.[7] In order to further validate these items we asked an upper staff member to assess the most important dimension, the ability to make decisions, for all patients in the study. A somewhat higher correlation ($\geq .8$) resulted from this comparison of assessment by upper staff and by nurses and aides.

We abstracted medical and demographic information from patient records after the observation was concluded. We coded a variety of variables including diagnoses, medications, ADL (activities of daily living) evaluations and sociodemographic data.

Case summaries for each patient and resident were written by coders after the data collection was complete. They followed a standard outline and included the types of observations and interviews done, general physical and mental conditions, summaries of staff ratings and ADLs, personal issues (eg, relationships with family members, preferences about living arrangements), and expected disposition. These summaries were directly available by computer during the analysis.

Informed Consent

Given that we were studying ethical issues, we found ourselves with an embarrassing difficulty obtaining meaningful informed consent from many of the skilled and intermediate patients and residents. Most of the patients were cognitively impaired.[8] Although we had little difficulty in obtaining consents from the few unimpaired patients (only one unimpaired patient approached for an interview refused), it was clear that most of the impaired patients were not able to understand the consent form, let alone make an informed decision about project participation. For example, comments made by one intermediate patient (after listening to an observer read and explain the consent form) suggested that she thought that she was being approached to have some work done on a house she used to own. Despite numerous explanations, other patients seemed unable to distinguish the observers from regular facility staff.

An alternative strategy was to obtain consent for observation of these patients from their family members. Many patients, however, had no families or had families who were not available. After some discussion, then, we decided to restrict our observations of patients who could not consent (and for whom we could not obtain proxy consent) to the dayroom and other public spaces. We did not interview any of these patients and we entered their rooms only once—while observing a staff member on medication rounds. To the best of our knowledge, patients voiced no discontent with our visit to their rooms or our presence in communal areas.

We ran into similar difficulty obtaining informed consent from residents, some of whom were also cognitively impaired (30% according to the staff ratings).[9] This surprised us, as cognitively impaired individuals were not supposed to be residing in this setting.

Again, we decided to interview only those residents who were clearly capable of informed decision-making and to supplement that data with staff interviews, record reviews, and observation of residents in communal areas.[10]

We also sought informed consent from each staff member of the facility who was likely to be observed or interviewed. Most staff agreed to participate and our ability to collect data from staff was, for the most part, not constrained. The upper staff of both the patient and resident settings, and the line staff of the residence, in particular, readily agreed to participate in the project. In fact, some staff not originally scheduled for interviews requested that they be interviewed.

The patient unit nurses and aides, however, were a little more hesitant about becoming involved in the project, although all except one eventually gave formal consent. These staff indicated that they were afraid that their comments would be shared with facility administration. We were able to allay staff fears somewhat by explaining the use of codes in place of names for staff, patients, and residents.

The larger issue, however, was the effect of organizational influences on staff consent, ie, did employees of this facility believe they had the option of saying no given that the project had the active support of their superiors? Our general impression is that they saw allowing the observers to be present as the lesser of two hazards—the greater hazard being angering their supervisors by resisting participation.

Overall, the nature of observations collected on the patient units suggests that most of these staff became accustomed to our presence, and—over time—many nurses and aides went out of their way to provide additional information to the observers. We came to feel that, with both staff and patients, our right to do the study was something that the observers earned over time rather than gained at the outset through the formal consent process.

Analysis

The analysis of our data was made easier and systematized by the use of the UNIX Text Analyst (UTA), a computerized review process that allows for the integration of qualitative and quantitative content analysis. What UTA does is to permit the analyst to see in rapid succession on the computer screen all places in the text that are marked with any specific code or series of codes. Moreover, the analyst's request to see portions of the text can be restricted or qualified by specifying a value for one or more of the nontext codes in the database provided that they in some way characterize a sector of the text (eg, the age of the speaker). For example, the analyst may ask to see all sections of text coded as "prohibitions" (one code we used), and then further limit the sections reviewed to instances in which the patient has been in the facility for more than a year and the speaker is an upper staff member. UTA will then show the particular speaker turn in question within the context of the entire observation. The analyst will see the selected speaker turn starred and in the middle of the screen. She will then be able to scroll back and forth around that turn to try to understand the context. When finished, the analyst can look at the next instance with a single keystroke. Brief descriptions of the speaker, the person spoken to, and the person being spoken about are available with a one-button command at any time.

The adaptation of this program for our research resulted in the linking of a database of conversational exchanges coded for content with all other relevant information. Through this approach, the meaning of a particular type of interaction could be explored in relation to auxiliary information, such as medical history, cognitive status, current medications, case disposition, staff ratings, ADL evaluations, and a variety of sociodemographic variables. This process circumvents some of the traditional limitations of both qualitative and quantitative approaches; it permits a more in-depth analysis than that provided by quantitative techniques alone, while providing a means by which analysts can consider all instances of a relevant topic within context rather than just those they remember.[11]

We began our analysis with a sequential reading of all 241 text files. These files consisted of transcribed verbatim accounts of conversations, observations, and taped semi-structured interviews obtained from staff, patients, residents, and families, as well as notes from discharge and planning meetings, care conferences, and admissions tours. Each file contained either a complete unit of information (eg, an interview, a meeting) or a series of observations of interactions made continuously during a particular time period. They averaged approximately eight pages in length and varied from one to fifty pages. By reviewing these files chronologically, we were able to note changes in patients and their relationships to others over time.

Next we developed a set of content codes for the textual data that reflected the issues of interest.[12] After a long series of discussions and preliminary coding, we settled on 62 codes subsumed under five general topics:

1. Aspects of the Setting (activities, time usage, financial considerations).
2. Roles and Behaviors (positive and negative evaluations by staff, patients or residents, and families).
3. Management (physical redirection and restraint, dissemination of information, aggression).
4. Interactions (requests by patients for assistance, permission, and information).
5. Issues of the Individual (respect for and violation of physical privacy norms, references to death and dying).

Following the line coding of all textual data, we prepared a summary of findings about each content code that featured excerpts from the text as examples supporting and countering our original hypotheses. These reviews were read and discussed, and modifications of the analyses were made (eg, some codes were collapsed and re-reviewed in combination). When completed, the most productive of these reviews were summarized, critiqued, and rewritten by each of the authors. These summaries of our empirical findings form the basis for the following chapters.

Conclusion

The goal of this project was to increase understanding of the various factors that affect the autonomy of persons living in long-term care facilities. We therefore chose to examine the daily lives of patients and residents in a fairly typical nursing home and residential living area. Participant observation was chosen as our methodology because of its ability to document, in extraordinary detail, the ways in which the institution affected the daily lives of participants. Interviews and more quantitative methods were utilized to supplement participant observation when necessary.

Before our findings are presented, several limitations need to be emphasized. First, all our data comes from the same general facility. While we have discussed our findings with many others who are involved with long-term care and they report similar observations, the generalizability of this data is problematic. Our findings should be treated as generating hypotheses that will require further confirmation.

Moreover, even within the facility, our methods were designed to produce insight rather than to generate systematic analyses. We might have increased the systematicity of our observations, but it would have been done at the expense of our understanding of the phenomenon. The result, then, is that statements about distributions should not be taken as rigorous findings. They are, at best, only general indicators of the population distributions. The above concerns notwithstanding, we are comfortable with the general validity of what follows.

NOTES

1. For an excellent introduction to the day-to-day lives of those living in long-term care settings, see Jaber Gubrium's *Living and Dying at Murray Manor*, New York: St. Martin's Press, 1975.

2. The third residential area floor was opened immediately prior to the start of data collection, and recruitment was ongoing during our stay.

3. While we observed a fairly steady turnover rate on skilled units (with patients transferred to rehabilitative facilities or another hospital, or discharged to home care), intermediate patients were seldom discharged. In fact, several had been living in intermediate care for more than ten years. During our data collection only four patients left the intermediate unit; three died, and the fourth was moved (at his request) to another facility.

4. Initial admission on the skilled units was determined almost exclusively by medical condition (ie, one or more conditions meeting the criteria for Medicare or Medicaid reimbursement). The various services provided to skilled patients for which this facility was reimbursed included post-operative recuperation for a wide variety of surgical procedures (such as repair of hip fractures), treatment of acute conditions (like systemic infections and uncontrolled diabetes), and time-limited rehabilitation (eg, physical therapy for stroke patients). Admission to intermediate care, on the other hand, depended primarily on the patients' (or families') ability to manage the costs of care (either through self-pay or insurance) and the patients' need for assisted living.. Although many of the intermediate patients that we observed had medical conditions similar to those of skilled patients, none of the former had medical conditions that met the criteria for skilled care. The conditions seen most frequently among intermediate patients included senile dementia, Parkinson's disease, hypertension (controlled), arthritis, and cardiovascular disease. The most frequent diagnoses for residents were hypertension, heart conditions, arthritis, and history of various forms of cancer. Surprisingly, seven of the residents had psychiatric diagnoses including schizophrenia, depression, agitated depression, and manic-depressive illness.

5. The data for this project was collected prior to the recent change in nursing home regulation that requires the formal certification of aides.

6. Since there were few upper staff members in this facility and usually not more than two holding any particular position, we tried to maintain their anonymity by referring to upper staff members diffusely as US—#. In a few places where it is essential for understanding the discussion, we have identified them by profession or position. The result is a delicate balance which we hope serves the values of both confidentiality and adequate reporting.

7. We believe that the poor correlation between nurse and aide ratings for this item resulted from the general exclusion of aides from meetings during which the involvement of families—particularly the involvement of families who did not live locally—in patient care decisions was discussed.

8. "Ability to make rational decisions independently" was scored by a nurse, an

aide, and an upper staff member (social worker) for each skilled and intermediate patient who participated in this study. Scoring ranged from 1 (no impairment) to 7 (complete impairment). At least one of the two line staff gave 74.2% of these patients a score equal to or greater than 4. Both of the two line staff gave 63.6% of these patients a score equal to or greater than 4. When the social worker's scores were substituted for the *lesser* of the two line staff scores, 81.8% of these patients received two scores equal to or greater than 4.

9. "Ability to make rational decisions independently" was scored by the residential nurse and a resident monitor for each resident who participated in our study. Scoring ranged from 1 (no impairment) to 7 (complete impairment). At least one staff member gave a rating of 4 or greater to 66.7% of the residents, while both gave a rating of 4 or greater to 30%.

10. All cognitively intact residents were approached for interviews. Most declined, citing such reasons as lack of interest in the project and busy schedules. It is also possible that they were unenthusiastic about involvement in a project that also involved skilled and intermediate patients. Despite the fact that patients and residents were housed under the same roof (albeit in different building wings), it was clear that residents disliked being identified with those individuals living on what they (residents) disparagingly referred to as "the other side."

11. Of course the same database could be explored through quantitative techniques. We chose not to do so because we felt that our data was not a representative sample of any population (eg, American nursing homes) and thus should not be used for the purpose of describing population parameters.

12. During the first few weeks of coding we conducted a series of inter-rater reliability checks on ten randomly selected files. Basically, we addressed two different, but related questions: (1) did the raters use the same number of codes per coded file, and (2) did the raters use the same content codes across all ten files? One-way analysis of variance indicated that there was no significant difference between the total number of codes used by coders per file, while a kappa coefficient ($k = .84$) indicated a high degree of reliability between coders relative to the specific content codes used. Overall, these statistics suggest little difficulty among coders in identifying and appropriately categorizing statements for content. Coding of speaker turns was based solely on their content with a maximum of six content codes assigned to each speaker turn. Each turn that contained one or more content codes was given a unique speaker code. Each code contained seven distinct types of information: the file name; the turn number; speaker, co-participant and other participant identification numbers; a context code, which categorized interactions by the setting or activity that was on-going (eg, music therapy); and a reference code, which identified the party being discussed. After developing specific rules for coding each line component, we began formal coding.

4

The Value Basis of Long-Term Care

Why do values matter? Certainly when we think about the autonomy of nursing home residents, we are concerned primarily with behaviors. We want to know how the staff promotes or undermines the patient's ability to form goals and to work toward them. We want to look at the behavior of the patients themselves to see to what degree their lives are self-controlled rather than lived at the initiative of others. Our focus is to concentrate on actual behavior, not theoretical values.

We might therefore begin by clarifying what we mean by "value." We are not talking, as an economist might, about things or states that are inherently desirable, ie, that have "objective" value. Rather we are referring to people's beliefs or conceptions of what is desirable. We are using the philosopher's notion of value as the private conception of what is desirable. Unlike the philosopher's typical description of how autonomous individuals develop their values, we believe that society, to a large degree, instills certain values into all of us. It is not random chance that leads Hindus to value different things than secular rationalists in the West. Likewise values are, to some degree, inherent in the roles that we adopt; they are socially structured.

Thus we define values as "conceptions of the desirable" (Parsons 1958). We hear them in the everyday discussions of staff, patients, and families. "Mrs. Jones needs to have her leg amputated" reflects health values just as the aide's disgusted reaction to a patient's leaving a mess on the floor reflects values of order and cleanliness. Yet why should we take these expressions of desirability seriously? Talk, as they say, is cheap. Are not what we are calling values basically just talk?

The problem with such a statement is contained in the "just." For it is through such "talk" that we justify to ourselves and others our patterns of activity. It is precisely such conceptions of desirable ends that we use to orient our behavior, and to justify to ourselves and others what we are trying to accomplish (Schutz 1967). The values that a group or institution professes to hold are the symbolic structures within which members of a group or institution coordinate activities and persuade other members to undertake certain activities.

In thinking about how one describes values, it is important to recognize that values differ by reference group. Thus a nurse, when talking with another nurse, may formulate her activity as directed toward improving nursing care quality. However, in the context of talking with an administrator, the desirability of filling beds may become the dominant value expressed in the discussion. It is easy to dismiss such "contradictions" as deception. The reality, however, is that we all hold a variety of values, many of which conflict in some situations. How these contradictory values are expressed and to whom is described in this chapter.

In analyzing the value structure of the nursing home setting we began by reviewing all statements that express approval or disapproval of someone's behavior. These evaluations of behavior provide us with a clear picture of the sorts of behavior that staff, patients, and family prefer, ie, how they think others ought to act. The data will be described in terms of whose behavior is being evaluated and who is doing the evaluation in order to determine if there are differences in values between the administrators, upper and lower staff, patients, and families in the nursing home.

Positive Staff Evaluations

Let us start with the positive evaluations that staff make of patients' behaviors.[1] These statements should illuminate the behaviors that staff approve of and wish to encourage. Even a quick look at this material reveals that the staff value autonomous behavior. While there are many examples of positive comments about patient and resident behavior that are not in any way related to autonomy, there are many which are. For example, in discussing one resident who refused a recommendation that she go to the hospital, an upper staff member commented:

> OBSERVER: Did Mrs. Walters (a resident) go into the hospital?
>
> UPPER STAFF–03: No, she stayed here. She refused to go to the hospital. She's very afraid that when she gets there, that she will not get

out. She's a smart lady, and she's probably right. Or she'll go to Psych again.

Comments about patient character that focused primarily on autonomy-related values were made frequently by staff. Thus patients were approvingly referred to as "active, "a fighter," "a self-sufficient one," "trying to keep her independence," and as having "dignity and self-esteem."

Of course the staff spoke approvingly about a wide range of patient behaviors, including incidents when patients behave passively. Consider the following discussion between a floor nurse, an aide, and the observer about a man who was admitted to the nursing home after having visited his wife there for a number of years.

> OBSERVER: What's with Mrs. Friedman?
> NURSE TAYLOR: It's nothing unusual. She's usually like this.
> MRS. DAWBER (AN AIDE): Yeah.
> OBSERVER: I heard that Mr. Friedman (her husband) is a concentration camp survivor.
> MRS. TAYLOR: Yeah. I also heard they lost all their family.
> OBSERVER: They don't seem to get along too well . . .
> MRS. TAYLOR: Huh!! It's a love and hate thing. Even before he became a patient here. (sounds disgusted)
> OBSERVER: How long ago was that?
> MRS. DAWBER: Oh, about a month ago.
> OBSERVER: And he visited her here before that?
> MRS. TAYLOR: Yeah, for at least six years. It's been hard for him. I mean getting used to being a patient here. But he has adjusted pretty well, hasn't he? (to Mrs. Dawber)
> MRS. DAWBER: Yeah.
> MRS. TAYLOR: He's really pretty nice. And he's had to take a lot lately.

Patients are also referred to approvingly as "taking all his meds," "a real gentleman," "never complains," "behaving better," etc. Sometimes the support both for autonomy and for more passive patient behavior came from the same staff person about the same patient:

> US–01: Lydia can be very difficult, but Lydia can be . . . I think that Lydia just doesn't want to lose her identity. She knows that she's a patient here, but she doesn't view herself as a patient. And that's good. I mean, you know, I understand what she's saying and where she's coming from. But, by the same token, she is a patient and she

does have to adopt certain institutional rules. And that's where Lydia gets hung up.

Sometimes positive statements were used as part of an effort to get patients to comply with staff desires. The following interaction occurred between a nurse and one of the patients who had been put on restricted access to the bathroom because she wanted to use it "every 10 minutes":

MRS. SILVERMAN: When do I go in?
US–04: I asked the aide. She said you just went in before dinner and you can go in again at 20 minutes to 7.
MRS. SILVERMAN: 20 of 7? (looking at watch) But it's been at least an hour or two.
US–04: No, Mildred. You were just in there before dinner. She'll come and take you in when it's time. You're doing real well on your schedule. (Her tone of voice is patronizing.)
MRS. SILVERMAN: (angrily) No, she won't! They do it when it's convenient for them!

Overall, the frequency of comments that seem supportive of autonomy and assertive activities were roughly equal to those that seem supportive of more passive behavior.

The above evidence seems, on the surface, to show substantial support among the staff for patient autonomy. However, a closer analysis shows that many of the statements supportive of autonomy are focused on residents (as we will see, the residence staff has a different "culture" than the nursing staff). The rest of the statements supporting autonomy come from the upper staff. There is not a single comment from the line staff (either aides, LPNs, or RNs) that reflects support for patient autonomy. Indeed, aside from approving comments about the compliance of particular patients, there are no positive comments at all about patients from line staff with the following exception:

NURSE BIGGS: It's not too bad . . . take Hilda Kramer for example. She has Parkinson's, but she likes to feed herself. And I don't care how messy it gets, as long as she likes to do it. As long as she wants to do it, she can do it.
OBSERVER: Hmm.
MRS. BIGGS: I think that is important, don't you?
OBSERVER: Yes, I do.
Observation: *I also think it's important, though, that the staff remain*

in the lounge area to help the patients during dinner. Mrs. Graves loses half of every meal, and sometimes ends up eating with her hands because her silverware is on the floor. Mrs. Kramer is often not given all of her meal. The rest is sometimes out of her reach and ends up being sent back to the kitchen. Further, she can use silverware instead of her hands if she is prompted to do so. Without that prompting, though, she generally uses her hands, smearing food all over herself and her geri-chair.

It should be obvious that the observer suspects the motives of the nurse's statement are based more on her desire to minimize work than on a genuine concern for autonomy.

Negative Staff Evaluations

Negative staff comments about patients are three times more frequent than positive ones.[2] Approximately two-thirds of the negative comments deal with patients who interrupt the staff-imposed structure with what the staff feel are unreasonable demands. These complaints can be subcategorized into three areas: concerns about order, responses to patient demands, and concerns about noncompliance with treatment regimens.

In all three areas, a common theme was heard: staff do not have time to adjust the care regimen to the particular peculiarities of individual patients. We will discuss the staff's desire for order in more detail later when we discuss the nursing home as a "total institution." For now it is important to see how this emphasis on institutional order leads staff to view independent patient behavior as interfering with proper care. Proper care is defined as meeting certain standards regarding a patient's physical health and safety, not in terms of individual patient wishes. For example, patients often keep food in their rooms. The staff, who were quite concerned with pest control, would often go into patients' rooms and throw the food out when the patient was not there. One would not think of doing such a thing to one's friends or neighbors but, in the context of the institutional requirement for order and sanitation, it seems to the staff to be not only acceptable but laudable.

Staff also frequently complained about the effect of inter-patient conflicts on the institutional order. When patients fought, either physically or verbally, an effort was usually made to isolate them from one another. The fact that the fighting parties were spouses or old friends did not change staff's response. While this behavior may reflect the value that both staff and patients place on peace, order, and physical well-being, isolation as a means of control seems more appropriate to children than to autonomous adults.

The priority of order in the institutional routine is clearest in the staff response to the particular demands of individual patients. It is important to note that, for individuals who are physically disabled (which all of these patients were to a greater or lesser degree), most expressions of individual autonomy involve making demands on someone else, usually the staff. Staff responses to such requests reflect their sense that such requests interfere with the staff's getting their work done:

> Note: *Observer enters staff lounge to find an on-going discussion.*
> NURSE: Do you want to contribute to the fund?
> OBSERVER: For what?
> NURSE: The fund to send Bernie (a particularly demanding patient) to the Jewish Home.
> OBSERVER: Sure.
> AIDE: Me, too. That would be worth a month's allowance.

This same patient becomes the subject of discussion later when he does move.

> Note: *Nurse Ross says Mr. Friedman left this morning to take up residence at the Jewish home. She says that she is sure he will be back.*
> MRS. ROSS: I said to him, "You'll say you want something and they won't get it for you fast enough and then your face will turn all red and then you'll have another stroke." (pause) He'll be back.

Another example of the reaction to patient demands:

> Observation: *Mrs. Baker, Dawber, Kennedy (aides) and Nurse Taylor are in the staff lounge. Nurse Taylor is writing in a chart. I go in and sit down. From the lounge we can hear Mrs. Zelkan yelling.*
> MRS. ZELKAN: Nurse! Nurse!
> MRS. TAYLOR: (mimicking) Nurse! Nurse!
> Observation: *The nurse then makes an obscene gesture. Everyone laughs.*

Such anger comes out relatively often in staff discussion of, and interaction with, patients who are "demanding" or "picky." It is not simply that the patient is requesting the staff person's time. The following discussion of another patient is indicative:

> NURSE BIGGS: I see that Lily is back.
> NURSE ROSS: Yeah, and she's not doing well. She's been running a temperature on and off, and she looks like death warmed over . . . . It might be best [if she passes away].
> MRS. LINLEY (an aide): Yeah.
> MS. LAUGHREN (an aide): Well, she can go tonight, but not until after 11:00.
> Observation: *Ms. Laughren goes off duty at 11:00. Everyone laughs.*
> NURSE ROSS: I can take care of her when she's sick like today. But when she's acting out, I just want to hit her. (The nurse shakes her fist.)

Such hostility is not confined to the line staff. "Non-cooperation" or violating the medical norm that patients should cooperate with treatment (Parsons 1951) is devalued by both the upper and line staff. The following conversation took place at one of the weekly discharge and planning meetings:

> PHYSICAL THERAPIST: I'm not sure, I'm not seeing much progress, I'm trying to . . .
> OCCUPATIONAL THERAPIST: Good luck! She does what she chooses. She won't even dress herself. She has her private duty nurse do it. That's why she is paying her.
> PHYSICAL THERAPIST: That's right, she doesn't cooperate in physical therapy either.

While it is true that these attitudes are primarily directed to negative assertive behaviors on the part of the patients, the values that encourage cooperation and passivity often get applied to patients whose only sin is wanting to do things their own way. We noted earlier that the upper staff used a variety of phrases as praise for autonomous patients (eg, "feisty"). Line staff, however, do not react to patient initiative in the same way:

> OBSERVER: I saw Mrs. Carl roll herself down the hallway. That's the first time I've seen her do that.
> AIDE: Fortunately, she's usually in a geri-chair. She's a feisty one. As sure as you tell her you don't want her to do something that's exactly what she does. We have some real feisty ones down there.

Family Values

If the line nursing staff is not very enthusiastic about patient autonomy, families are not much more so. While our data on family values is limited,[3] our interviews show that family members are ambivalent about the value of autonomy. On the one hand, their reminiscences about family members prior to entry into the nursing home are replete with references to their competence and independence. Thus:

> I don't know. She's an independent person. And she's always been like that. I think she was very independent at an age when it wasn't "the great thing to be." She was walking to a different drummer maybe. But I think she used to be admired for that at that point in time as I look back over it. Not too many people could live by themselves at that point in time and live to be 80 and do everything.

Likewise, the families are supportive of efforts to regain an independent life style. Thus, they repeatedly express their support for physical therapy efforts and are critical if their relatives do not work at rehabilitation. In these cases it is not autonomous decision-making that is valued, rather the support is for a goal that the family thinks that the patient ought to value. Thus:

> I think she got to it. At that point she gave up, frankly. And would no longer push. As you have impairments you have to push to overcome them and she quit.

Another patient's daughter expressed the converse experience with her father, praising him for his enthusiasm:

> He was highly motivated and he was just the opposite and begging them to take him to therapy. He worked very hard and there was no question that he worked as hard as he could work. But again he hit a plateau, and his time ran out . . .

In spite of these positive evaluations of independence both on the outside and vis-à-vis physical therapy, there was little support for autonomous behavior on the units. Families, like the staff, valued compliance with the norms of the institution and placed the patient's physical well-being above attempts at individualization. Repeatedly the families criticized the patients as stubborn and uncooperative with staff or expressed pleasure at cooperation. One patient's child described her mother as independent and stubborn all her life but:

> I just think she is just there. And she does whatever you tell her at this point. And she might say "no I don't want to do it." But her negativism is just a carry-over from how she lived before. It was easy to say no and have nobody push you to do anything. I think that might be ingrained in there. But, she goes wherever they take her, which, I am flabbergasted that she does that. So I'm very pleased with how they care for her.

Indeed, in one instance, the patient's independence is cited as a reason for deciding that he had to be restricted:

> I'm appreciative of the nursing home's concerns. He isn't very stable. At this point in time I don't believe he's ambulatory at all. But going back two to three years, they were concerned that he would fall and hurt himself. So they preferred to keep him confined. And as I say he is a fighter. If they'd teach him to take two steps, he'd try to take ten. So we had a little give and take on that.

Residence Staff Values

We noted earlier that while the intermediate care staff and family value physical well-being and focus on the maintenance of unit order, the residence staff is considerably different.[4] Their complaints about resident behavior reflect their assumption that residents should be more, not less, autonomous. Consider the following comment by a residential nurse concerning a resident whom she did not think belonged there.

> NURSE MILLER: She was a very dependent person before she came in here. Very dependent. (with emphasis) She won't do anything for herself. She wouldn't even comb her hair if I didn't make her. She'll only make her bed if I tell her that she has to. (pause) This isn't the place for her.
> OBSERVER: Where would be an appropriate place for her?
> MRS. MILLER: I don't know. (pause) I guess intermediate care would be more right in a sense. (pause) She constantly walks and she needs a place for that. She's not incontinent and she feeds herself . . . (pause) It's her restlessness and her desire to be dependent on some-

> one else . . . They (intermediate care) can provide for that over there.

While the residence nurse notes that the patient meets two of the formal qualifications for living on the residential side (qualifications that some other residents she values do not meet), her assertion that the resident does not belong emphasizes the importance she places on autonomy.

The limits of the monitors' sense of entitlement to direct the residents' lives is most clear in those cases in which they disapprove of specific behaviors. The monitors often express ambivalence about behavior that, although autonomous, seems misguided.

> MS. BLACK (a resident monitor): Yeah. You know . . . they are all adults and they are all responsible for their own thing. We're just here to monitor. It may upset us a lot to see how they're throwing their time away. We have activities that we encourage them to go to. I can name some that will not go even if you stand on your head. They choose to stay in their little rooms.
> OBSERVER: Will they read or watch TV?
> MS. BLACK: Sometimes not even that. Kathryn will not go to activities. I have said, "They are playing bingo downstairs." She'll say that she doesn't like bingo. I'll tell her to just go and be with other people. "You know, I wouldn't go and play bingo either. But why don't you go down?" And she'll just say, "No, I don't think so." She goes occasionally. And she may go to the movies. Or walk. I'll have one of the girls from recreation call and say, "Come get Kathryn." Her attention span and her train of thought does not stay long. Sometimes she just walks out of places. She doesn't even watch television. A couple of our ladies watch television and fall asleep, but Kathryn will not even join them. She's Catholic, and on Sunday they will bring communion around. And I'll say, "The ladies are joining together for communion. Why don't you join them?" She'll say, "I don't think I'll go down." So there. It upsets me that she doesn't fill up her day more, or participate more but that's what she chooses and she's allowed to do that. We're not a prison or a real structured . . . We encourage them.

The monitors also complain about residents who are too demanding of their time. Like the intermediate care line staff, they object to spending their time tending to patient demands. However, the tone of such complaints is markedly different. Instead of suggesting that their charges should not want things, they imply that the residents should do the things themselves.

> NURSE MILLER: See, like downstairs. There's this lady who sits at a table for four. I won't mention her name. And she came to me and she said, "I don't see why I have to sit at that table with a woman who passes gas." Well, I could understand that. I mean, she was trying to eat and all. So I moved her over to another table. She was really wound up about it. And then, the next day, she called me over to her table and she stuck her finger in my face and said, "I don't think that I should have to sit over here away from my friends." I said, "You asked me to move you." And she said, "But I don't want to sit away from my friends." And I said, "I'm not going to move that other woman. She's sitting there with her friends, and they're not complaining about her. You were the one who asked to be moved." You see, they just won't try to solve their own problems. She wouldn't talk to the lady at the table who was passing gas. That lady didn't even know that there was a problem. They just try to pull us in the middle of it all. They won't tell you no, but they'll come and complain to us.

The resident monitors, although some of their charges differ only marginally from some of the intermediate care patients, complain in ways that reflect positive evaluations of resident autonomy. Indeed, their discussions of residents' care show strong similarities to the ethical literature on autonomy in the elderly. The following monitor might as well have been deliberately exemplifying Collopy's (1986) ideas about positive and negative autonomy.

> MRS. MCCULLOUGH (a resident monitor): She sleeps. From what I've seen of her, all she does is sleep. I feel that they need more activities. They just go in their rooms and sit there. It's making them worse.
> OBSERVER: How is it making them worse?
> MRS. MCCULLOUGH: Because they're regressing inside themselves. Jessie's a perfect example of that. They really need to be pushed to go do things. You know, go for a walk or do something.
> OBSERVER: What if they just want to veg? Like Mr. Detrich? Is that OK?
> MRS. MCCULLOUGH: I would say it's OK. They have that right. But if you let them veg all of the time, they're going to be a veg sooner or later. If you don't keep that mind going, you have nothing.
> OBSERVER: How do you put that across to somebody like Mr. Detrich?

MRS. MCCULLOUGH: "Get up and go!! Jessie, you have to go." Or he will not.

Conclusion

In summary, the value patterns of family and staff are strangely parallel. Both groups strongly support autonomy and there is no reason to believe that this belief is not genuine. On the contrary, we were struck that for the upper staff the commitment to autonomy was basic to their conceptions of themselves as professionals. Likewise, the family members spoke with genuine pride of the independence and strength of character of their parents. Yet the approval of autonomy seems to stop at the nursing home door. The floor staff that actually was responsible for the patient's daily life could find little to praise about patients except when they passively cooperated. They saw most manifestations of autonomy as unreasonable demands. Likewise, families seemed to feel that cooperation and passivity were the appropriate behaviors from their nursing home bound relatives. Both groups saw physical well-being as a more important value in the nursing home situation than autonomy.

The ethos of the residential side was quite different. The caregivers here viewed promoting autonomy as central to their role. Autonomous behavior, rather than constituting a problem, was one of the primary goals of residential living. This difference between the intermediate care facility and the residential living quarters will arise again in other chapters and will constitute an important finding of our study.

NOTES

1. Keeping with our general feeling that we have a special sample and that statistics would not be meaningful, we have not provided percentages of occurrences of various types in our field notes. However, in order to indicate the size of the data from which we are generalizing, we will provide the number of instances of each type of interaction that we discuss. There were 65 occurrences of staff making positive comments about patient behaviors.

2. There were 215 instances of staff making negative comments about patients.

3. There are 36 instances of family members making favorable comments about patients' behaviors and 51 negative comments.

4. There are 57 positive staff statements about residents' behaviors and 154 negative statements.

5

Caring and Cared-for: Role Relationships in Long-Term Care

Humans do not interact with each other simply as people. We conduct our activities in role relationships. Whatever we know about and feel for our parents or our children, we relate to them in the context of the parent-child relationship. Likewise patients in a nursing facility are not known by the staff simply as human beings, but as patients. The patients do not know the staff simply as a collection of people, but as members of the staff. Our task in this chapter is to explore the meaning of the role relationship of staff and patient and its impact on patient autonomy.

The nursing home section of the facility that we studied was clearly intended to be thought of as a medical facility. This fact was essential to understanding the nature of the relationships in the nursing home and affected the patients' ability to live autonomously in the nursing home setting.

The emphasis on medical care was made clear in a variety of subtle and not-so-subtle ways. The individuals who lived in this setting were referred to by staff as "patients." Patients' identities as patients dominated almost everything else about them. Staff frequently referred to patients as "that patient" or by their medical condition. Another variation on this was identification by unit (eg, skilled vs intermediate). In the following excerpt, for example, staff members try to decide which patients should remain on the intermediate unit following music therapy. Unlike some of the previous examples where the patients were identified by name, staff in this example do not use names to distinguish between patients.

US–13: Who else goes? (to a skilled floor)
Observation: *US–13 and Mrs. Linley (an aide) look across the remaining patients.*
Mrs. Linley: That's the only odd one I see. That one. (pointing)
US–13: OK.
Observation: *US–13 rolls the unidentified "odd" patient over to the visitor elevator.*

Patients were often no more differentiating about staff than staff were about patients. Patients saw the facility as a primarily medical institution; many referred to all of the staff as "nurse," irrespective of training. For example, in spite of considerable efforts at explanation, our female observer was sometimes called "nurse" even though she wore street clothes and provided no nursing care. Patients seemed either unable or disinterested in making any distinctions between the different staff members who cared for them.

In addition, the intermediate care unit's environment was reminiscent of a hospital ward. Most of the staff wore the white uniforms characteristic of nurses and hospital aides. The physical layout also was modeled after a hospital ward—long corridors with flanking rooms. (Perhaps this should not have been surprising since the facility was a hospital that had been converted to a nursing home.) Likewise the furniture looked like it had been purchased from a hospital supply house. Staff kept medical records in a format that was clearly borrowed from hospital record-keeping. Medications were passed out off a cart in the same manner that they typically are in a hospital.

These observations are, of course, completely unremarkable. In another sense, however, they are of central importance as they convey to all concerned that this was a medical facility and therefore generated certain expectations. The initial path of our analysis will be to describe the medical role model in general, and to show how it affected the role expectations in the nursing home component of the facility. We will then contrast this with the residential area, a nonmedicalized setting, and consider how the very different situational definition and role expectations led to different role relationships.

The Role Relationships of Patient and Physician

While physicians play a relatively minor role in the care and management of the patients in the nursing facility, the social expectations guiding the doctor-patient relationship are central to our understanding of the role the elderly assume in the nursing home. A dominant feature of a culturally defined patient role is the need for help (Parsons 1951). Patients are seen as representing deviance from the culturally defined ideal of physical well-being, a condition for which they are not held responsible, but for which they are assumed to need assistance. While the patient is not responsible for being ill, however, she is responsible both for getting help and for following the physician's recommendations. If she fails to do so, it is appropriate (even expected) for family, friends, and health care professionals to use sanctions to change her behavior. It is important to note that illness is not something that the layperson defines for herself. Instead, it is ultimately up to the physician to certify the appropriateness of an illness claim or, if necessary, impose the definition on a patient who does not seek the role.

Moreover, the sick role assumes that the necessary help cannot be provided by the patient or other laypersons, but must be obtained from designated health care professionals. The inability of the patient both to determine the nature of the problem and to choose the scientifically best treatment is seen as justifying the view that the sick person must rely on the health professional's judgment to determine the appropriate course of action. More specifically, patients must cede authority to health care professionals for what is normatively defined as out of their control.

This conceptualization of the patient's role and its ethical import has been the subject of intense discussion by medical ethicists over the last two decades (Katz 1984, Faden and Beauchamp 1986, Appelbaum et al 1987). We have already reviewed some of this in our discussion of the importance of autonomy in medical ethics (Chapter 1) and we will not repeat it here. However, it seems important to note that this description of the patient's role seems to fit best the acutely ill patient. When the patient is suffering acutely or in need of emergency help, for example, the physician must act with little input from the patient. For the chronically ill patient, this abdication of responsibility signifies not just a loss of autonomy for a specific event, but a loss of control over a significant component of his life (Lidz et al 1985). The implications of this view for the autonomy of nursing home patients is apparent when one analyzes the role relationships in the intermediate and the skilled care settings.

Role Relationships in Intermediate and Skilled Care

The role relationships between patients and professional caregivers (from physicians to aides) within the nursing home drew heavily from the normative structure of the doctor-patient relationship. Health care professionals conceptualized their primary obligation as acting to maximize patients' health, in particular their physical well-being. Patients, on the other hand, were expected to attempt to get better by complying with health care professionals' recommendations. This emphasis is clear in numerous examples of interviews and routine conversations among staff. For example, in response to a quite global question about possible caregiving improvements within the institution, an upper staff member volunteered suggestions solely related to physical well-being:

> US–03: . . . things like mouthcare. I'm not saying that it's not done. I'm saying that it is not done as frequently as it should. Cleaning your teeth, cleaning your gums, rinsing our mouth out . . . . Feet-care. These are two of the things that are left for last because it is easier to help get someone up when they need help than to do these other things. Then you can move on to somebody else. The major things are never left undone. They're (institution staff) really quite good about major components of care.

Within this general staff focus on care, the primary emphasis appears to relate almost exclusively to traditional medical care of the body—with a primary focus on acute care of remediable biomedical diseases. This focus is pervasive and is reflected in a wide variety of institutional rituals and procedures. For example, at the discharge and planning meetings (at which most of the substantial decisions about patient care were made), a particular upper staff member would routinely present the case for consideration by the other staff members. The way in which cases were presented reflected what upper staff saw as essential information that needed to be considered in making plans. A typical example follows:

> US–01: OK, this is Wilma Brown. She is 54, and this is her second admission here. She was home just one day, fell, and fractured her hip. She also had multiple other problems including a skin disease, congestive heart failure, COPD (chronic obstructive pulmonary disease), a deep venous thrombosis (clot in leg), and so on.

This medicalization of the patient does not appear to have been specific to upper staff but, rather, crossed staff lines. Among line staff (registered and practical nurses and aides), the medicalization of tasks was commonly reflected in a preference for acute care over custodial care (ie, basic support for activities of daily living).

> OBSERVER: Is it better here than at other places where you've worked?
> NURSE BIGGS: Uh-huh. Absolutely. It's the way this center is set up. Some parts of it are still really acute care oriented, and that's the really good part about this place.

The emphasis on physical well-being and its expression in lower staff's preference for acute care did not go unnoticed by upper staff. In the following example, an upper staff member notes that this preference for acute, as opposed to custodial, care was pervasive.

> US–03: . . . even in a system like [the institution]. Long-term care isn't a part of their whole health care system. You'd be surprised at the mentality. It's like acute care is [the preference]. That's the thing in health care. You don't want to think about long-term care.

This preference was also observed in staff-patient interactions across various staff levels. In general, while staff responded to the relatively rare situations necessitating acute care with enthusiasm, they showed less interest in routinely assisting patients with activities of daily living and almost no interest in promoting patients' development of autonomous interests. This appeared particularly true with reference to the intermediate patient unit, where the majority of care could be accurately described as custodial in nature.

In the following example, an intermediate care charge nurse expresses her feelings about having to help prepare a patient for bed.

> Observation: *An unidentified aide rolls the new patient (Mr. Borza) down the hallway. Nurse Biggs gets up from her chair in the staff room and follows. They roll the patient to his room.*
> MRS. BIGGS: And we've got to put this monster (Mr. Borza) to bed?
> AIDE: Yes.
> MRS. BIGGS: Look at him! He's disgusting!
> Observation: *The patient in question is an elderly white man. He appears to be in his late seventies or early eighties. He is lying on a gurney, dressed only in a hospital gown. He appears to be completely "vegged out."*

Caregiving, then, was defined primarily as providing medical assistance, preferably acute care, and to a lesser degree, attention to activities of daily living. Custodial tasks (feeding, toileting, bathing) and individual attempts to help patients accomplish their goals were responded to, at best, without enthusiasm and, at worst, with anger and resentment.

While the staff's focus was clearly on care of the body, this interest did not seem to extend to the rehabilitative work necessary for the recovery of lost skills or the development of new skills. While medical techniques designed to prolong life were commonly used, techniques focused on informal rehabilitation (eg, walking patients on the unit, encouraging patients to do as much for themselves as they could) and the subsequent increase in patient autonomy were not. This was apparently seen as the responsibility of the Physical Therapy Department and not part of the unit care tasks. For example, in order to help her husband improve his functional status as much as possible after a hip fracture and subsequent illness, one patient's wife was forced into a running battle with the staff.

> OBSERVER: So he came back home from the hospital?
> MRS. ANDERSON (patient's wife): Well, no. [He was at a] nursing home at first for three or four weeks.
> OBSERVER: And stayed there and then came back here and that's when he started walking?
> MRS. ANDERSON: Yes. . . . They (staff) were very antagonistic to me when we went into [the institution].
> OBSERVER: In what sort of way?
> MRS. ANDERSON: I've never met a thing like that. Apparently, I walked into a hot potato situation that wasn't of my making. They were all very sensitive. Anything you asked about you would get back. You were wrong.
> OBSERVER: Can you think of a particular example?
> MRS. ANDERSON: Well, everything. I wanted to get him walking. I wanted him to have therapy. They said that he couldn't possibly handle their therapy program. He wasn't in good enough shape. I said, "Couldn't he walk?" And they said, "That would take three people. We don't have that much staff. We can't afford to spend three people walking him up and down the hall." First I said I could do it. They said, "You couldn't possibly do it." I said, "I've done it before. I brought him back. I can do it." So I went in and got him out of the chair. Nobody helped me. They didn't help me get him out of the geri-chair, which is a big heavy thing, I could hardly handle them. They just watched me. Antagonistic was the word. I don't know. . . . Finally they decided that the therapist would walk with him three times a week. That was wonderful. I had thought of it every day. Always wanting more. I said, "Don't they ever walk any of these

> people?" I was talking to the social service worker and the nurse. I said, "This isn't just your problem and my problem. This is the problem of the whole elder society who are in nursing homes. They're turning into vegetables. And I think something should be done about it." And I began to get a little action. Once in a while they'd walk with him. Now they're walking him twice a day.

Unfortunately, the staff's preferred goal of a broad-based patient recovery could not be realized due to the progressive nature of patient dementia. Most of the staff's time was spent not on acute care, but on the more mundane custodial tasks of helping patients get out of bed, go to the bathroom, and eat their meals. Staff were further frustrated by the increasingly burdensome custodial care required by cognitively deteriorating patients. The stress inherent in being unable to provide restorative care, staff's dislike of custodial duties, and the emotional distress caused by caring for cognitively impaired patients may be the explanation for many of the volatile patient-caregiver interactions seen both in this chapter and in later sections. Staff discontent with nonrestorative responsibilities was often directed toward the individuals for whom custodial care was necessary. In the following instance an intermediate unit aide reacts to finding some overturned paper cups and shredded tissues on the television lounge table.

> MRS. BAKER (an aide): Look at this mess! You people are disgusting! What are you doing!
> Observation: *She picks up all the shredded Kleenex and starts back down the hallway.*
> MRS. BAKER: Nancy (an aide)! Get some alcohol and come down here! This table has got to be cleaned up before the food gets here!
> OBSERVATION: *She storms back down the hallway and into the kitchenette.*

Staff resented the dependency of patients concerning the custodial tasks. Some patients were aware of the staff's attitude and felt that it resulted in their receiving inferior treatment:

> Observation: *Mrs. Bennett turns herself around and rolls herself down the hallway.*
> OBSERVER: Are you going to bed?
> MRS. BENNETT: I can't. God only knows when they (staff) are going to put me to bed.

There are many other comments in the data that indicate that staff found their cognitively impaired charges to be less than ideal human beings. In the following example the nurse is partly joking but the metaphor of contamination is strong:

> Observation: *The aide goes back down the hall. I tell Nurse Dawber that I'll be passing out cookies during the afternoon.*
> MRS. DAWBER: How are you going to do it?
> OBSERVER: I thought I would just leave trays of them in the TV lounge for those who can help themselves, and then go room to room for the others.
> MRS. DAWBER: Oh, I don't think you should do that. (seriously) (referring to leaving cookies in the lounge) You don't know where their (patients) hands have been. (pause) Unless I can have mine first. Then I don't care. (laughing)

The other major implication of staff's acceptance of the medical model was their expectation that patients would defer to them regarding medical decisions. Patients were expected to cooperate with all recommendations relating to what the staff defined as medical care.

In the following example, an upper staff member and the charge nurse are reinserting a patient's naso-gastric tube. The patient had repeatedly expressed her desire that the tube be removed and, when ignored, had removed it herself. On telephoned physician's orders, the tube was reinserted.

> Observation: *I walk down the hallway. As I pass room 3012 I can hear choking and gagging. The nurse had told me earlier that Mrs. McClain had pulled her ng tube out. I can hear US–04's voice. Apparently they are trying to reinsert it. It doesn't sound like it's going well.*
> US–04: Don't fight it, dear. (more choking and gagging) You're doing good. (more choking and gagging)

Most patients accepted the parameters of these role relationships. As noted above, patients also viewed the nursing home primarily as a medical institution. In general, patients exemplified the traditional patient role—they passively accepted health care professionals' assessments and followed their orders.

This behavior earned praise from staff:

> Observation: *We go into the small television lounge. Mr. Breese is sitting there.*
> NURSE DAVIES: Hello, Herbert.

MR. BREESE: (gibberish)
MRS. DAVIES: Put your eyes back. I'm going to put some drops in.
Observation: *The nurse puts some drops in his eyes. Mr. Breese winces.*
MRS. DAVIES: Good job. Very good job, Herbert.

Patients were encouraged by family members to cooperate with staff recommendations. The following comments suggest that families were concerned about the negative ramifications (to patients) of noncompliance.

> MRS. ANDERSON: (reconstructing conversation with her husband) "You ought to cooperate with them. You don't want to be difficult to get along with. You'll get better care if you cooperate."

Not all patients, however, agreed with these expectations, and some systematically failed to cooperate. The following example concerns a patient's response to being force-fed a medication by a nurse. Medication on this unit was commonly administered to demented patients by crushing it into ice cream.

Observation: *Nurse Taylor brings a container of ice cream to a patient sitting in front of the TV. The ice cream contains crushed medication. The nurse takes a spoonful of the ice cream and tries to put it in Mrs. Wingate's mouth. The patient appears to refuse to open her mouth. Nurse Taylor then drops the spoon back into the ice cream.*
MRS. TAYLOR: Then you eat it. (angrily)
Observation: *The nurse leaves the ice cream on the table and leaves the television lounge. She walks back down the hallway. Mrs. Wingate watches her leave. . . . Mrs. Wingate picks up the spoon and begins to eat the ice cream.*

Other more cognitively intact patients were able to articulate their feelings about the expectations that staff enforced.

OBSERVER: What do you not like about this place?
MRS. DUNN: Nonrecognition. That's the only thing that I can tell you about it.
OBSERVER: By the staff, you mean?
MRS. DUNN: Yeah. I don't think that they bother or care.

Another intact patient felt that patients were deprived of individual identities.

> Note: *Miss Kosak has mentioned that staff are disrespectful to patients.*
> OBSERVER: How are they disrespectful?
> MISS KOSAK: Well, they don't respect people as . . . They dehumanize people. "This one, this one, this one . . . go to bed." They don't ask if you want to go to bed, or if you'd like to stay up a little longer. . . . A lot of these people . . . they (staff) just manipulate them. I hate to see people manipulated. You know . . . to the chair . . . to the bed . . . then back to the chair. And that's all their lives consist of. And they (staff) decide where you're going to be at a certain time. I don't like that. They're still human beings. I think they should be asked if they want to do it. I feel that if I get like that, and I pray to the good Lord that I won't, that he'll take me. Because it's just like an assembly line at night. This one goes to bed and that one goes right down the line.
> OBSERVER: So it feels like an assembly line?
> MISS KOSAK: I'm not on an assembly line. "Don't treat me like that! I'm a person."
> OBSERVER: Do you tell them that?
> MISS KOSAK: I told them that. I said, "Don't treat me like I'm on an assembly line because I'm not." That's why they don't like me.

Attempts by patients to take a more active role were not viewed favorably by staff.

> US–03: Mrs. Owen's room is on one side of the hall. Adjacent to her room was a man by the name of Mr. White. And there was another guy in his room. And both of them (both of these guys have died since) didn't know how to use a call button. So they'd call out or yell. And Mrs. Owen would be like their advocate. "Nurse, you get down here. Why, he shouldn't have to lay."
> OBSERVER: Did the staff take it in good humor or did they get ticked off?
> US–03: No. I think they were ticked off about it. I really do. I don't think they saw it as being therapeutic for Mrs. Owen to be able to just literally stick up . . . for somebody else in need.

In summary, we found that both staff and patients recognize a defined role for patients, characterized by compliance and cooperation rather than autonomous self-direction. While not all patients accepted this role, in practice it dominated all other patient roles. While there was some discomfort with these role relations on both sides, there was little or no effective challenge to the traditional health care provider-patient relationship. While the doctor-patient relationship is generally thought of as a warm if paternalistic one, the adoption of this model in the nursing home led to anger and stress.

Role relationships in the nursing home, however, were not exclusively focused around the patient-staff relationships. Unlike most medical care for adults, families are often deeply involved in long-term care. Thus, in order to understand the context within which patients are or are not able to act autonomously, we need to look at both the role of the family as defined by staff and the role of the staff as defined by family members. To put it another way, we need to look at how each party defined the other vis-à-vis their respective roles with patients.

Family Roles

One of the more important roles that staff expected families to assume was helping with the routine custodial care of their relatives. However, their moralism extended beyond self-interest. They thought family members should want to care for relatives. Some family members seemed more than willing to assume responsibility for their patient's custodial care. The family member cited below, for example, visited her mother almost daily and insisted on assuming responsibility for most of her needs that extended beyond the medical realm.

> DAUGHTER: They (staff) are so good and kind and loving to the patients here. . . . I'm just so glad to have her. (reference to patient) She's 94 now. And she's probably more hale and hearty than before. It's just remarkable. They take such wonderful care of them.

Family members who accepted this role responsibility, like the one above, were viewed by the staff as "good families" and received considerable staff support and approval.

> US–02: . . . Mrs. Graham. She had her sister, Elsie, up on six. She came in two or three times a week, taking two buses, and visited her sister. She'd bring magazines in. She'd talk with her. She was unbelievable as a visitor.

Of course the staff had a self-interest in assuring such normative behavior from family members. When family members helped with the custodial care this saved the staff from having to do the work.

Some families preferred that the staff assume responsibility for all aspects of care. Indeed, some families rarely or never visited. Families who were not as involved in aspects of custodial care as staff felt they should be were frequently the subject of disapproval.

> NURSE WALKER: (standing in doorway) Excuse me. Mr. Anderson's wife is here. He's not poseyed. She said she'll let us know when she leaves.
> Observation: *Mrs. Walker leaves.*
> NURSE ROSS: It'll be at dinner time.
> MRS. CHAMBERS (an aide): Yeah, she'll be out of the door like a shot.
> OBSERVER: Why?
> MRS. ROSS: So she won't have to feed him.
> MRS. CHAMBERS: Yeah. (nods her head in agreement)

The staff and family sometimes disagreed about the staff's conceptualization of their role. These disagreements centered on three topics. First, as noted above, staff viewed themselves as medical professionals and were therefore least interested in providing chronic rehabilitative therapies. Some families expressed dissatisfaction with this approach.

> DAUGHTER: They (staff) have 35 patients. (per unit) Just so they wash, . . . feed them, get them cleaned up from breakfast, ready for lunch, take them down to whatever activities they are going to, bring them back up, give them dinner . . . I really don't find fault there. But things that they don't seem to think about . . . [what is] beyond the next task . . . at [the institution]. All they really seem to be geared towards is that they take care, excellent care of the patients, but they don't think about how to encourage a person to do more for themselves.

Still, most families tended to agree with the staff about their role responsibilities. They saw this focus on physical care as part of the institutional setting.

> WIFE: It's just very hard to get anything like that (focus on mental stimulation) done in a nursing home. I think that it goes back to the base that therapy took care of everything. Anything physical. All they (staff) did was take care of the people physically. Actively is what I mean. The nurses and aides were accustomed to taking care of their (patients) bodily needs.

A more common conflict was over what constituted appropriate care of the body. Families often objected to what they perceived as the failure to provide what they saw as a minimum of care, particularly custodial care.

> WIFE: Well, I'd like them (staff) to take him (husband) to the bathroom regularly. He was not incontinent. He probably is now, because every time I'd come in, he wanted to go to the bathroom. They were very impatient. They'd say, "Well, he has a diaper on." And I said, "Well, actually he doesn't need the diaper if you would take him to the bathroom."
> OBSERVER: So how come he had the diaper?
> WIFE: They just diaper people. They say, "What are we going to do if he has to go to the bathroom while we're serving supper?"

In a few cases, family members did their best to force staff into assuming responsibility for activities of daily living and were conceptualized (by upper staff, at least) as having some negotiating power.

> US–03: But they (families) don't want to hear about it. They don't want to hear that you forgot to put dentures in. They don't want to hear that you haven't sat somebody on the commode. . . . We have to extend ourselves even more because those families are paying big money to have their family member here. And that's the bottom line.

Finally, conflicts arose concerning the family's role in medical decision-making. Periodic conflict between staff and family suggests that some families had trouble with the role that staff assigned to them, ie, cooperation with staff treatment decisions and the providing of auxiliary assistance. As shown in the example below, families appeared to expect more collaboration in decision-making:

> DAUGHTER: And there was another time where he (father) said he was having chest pains and they (nursing home staff) were all ready to send him to (hospital) and I said, "Wait a minute. Don't send him until I get there." So I went over there and said, "Dad, is anything hurting you?" I was called and they said you were having chest pains. And all he said was, "I just want to get out of here." So he was faking chest pains. The nurses wouldn't believe me. . . . She (one nurse) said to me, "Your father could been having a heart attack . . ." Then the doctor the next day laughed about the whole thing. He thought it was hilarious and he said she was just doing her job. From her point

> of view [I was] a negligent family member who was trying to tell her how to do her job. . . . But . . . the response on that part of the staff was that maybe I was trying to keep my dad from getting care. That was pretty upsetting. That was one of the most upsetting experiences that I had.

Despite these minor variations, staff, patient, and family roles within this setting can be accurately described as an extension of the traditional doctor-patient model. Further, in spite of occasional disagreement with this approach by family, the majority of families appeared to accept these roles. Even those families who identified what they felt were negative facets of care, eg, the prominent concern with care of the body, were unwilling, for the most part, to directly challenge the staff authority.

The struggles that occurred between family members and staff about their respective roles did not appear to extend to conflicts over the patient's role. Conflicts centered largely around who would provide the auxiliary aspects of care, rather than the goals of care or the patient's role in the institution. Family members conceptualized the patient role in much the same way as the staff did. This has significant ramifications since, to the degree that the staff's actions are a response to extra-staff demands, the families (with a few exceptions) did not seem to be influencing the staff in the direction of promoting patient autonomy.

Role Relationships in the Residence

The intermediate and skill staff's primary emphasis on acute medical care, and its ramifications for patient's autonomy, did not appear to extend to the residential area. Residential monitors who, like the intermediate and skilled aides occupied the bottom of the ladder in their unit, valued independence and self-determination among the residents, and did their best to facilitate and encourage those types of behaviors. The protection and encouragement of self-determination among the residents by resident monitors appeared to be part of their conceptualization of their role.

> Resident Monitor Olson: I'm here to help them retain what little independence they still have. That's the only way I can describe it. If they need me to help them do something, I do it. But not take it away from them. If they're still able to move those extremities . . . even if it is messed up, but they're trying, they still feel that they did it

> themselves. You don't want to take that away from them. That's what I feel I'm here for—to help them retain what little bit they still have.

This basic philosophy extended to monitors' evaluation of residents' behavior. In the following example, a monitor expresses approval of the behavior of one of the more independent residents.

> RESIDENT MONITOR JONES: Then we have Mrs. Tataglia. She's 96. An Italian lady. Now there's a self-sufficient one. Oh, my. You get her towels ready and she gets in that tub and bathes herself . . . .
> OBSERVER: She sounds like the type of person the unit was designed for.
> MS. JONES: If I would put an apron on her, she would run the vacuum and dust the furniture. She's a typical mother. We do very little for Sophia. And then she'll start yelling at these people. "All you do is sit. Exercise! Exercise! Walk! Walk!"

Staff routinely encouraged residents who at least made attempts at self-sufficiency.

> Note: *The conversation pertains to a resident who alternated between cooperation and noncooperation relative to self-care.*
> RESIDENT MONITOR JOHNSON: . . . his memory. Long-term is good, but his short-term . . . No. And it depends upon how he feels about things that day. Sometimes he has an attitude where, "I don't care." And other times he makes an effort. He'll get up and say, "Good morning," and, "I made my bed." "You made your bed!!" (says monitor) "I'm shaving." (resident) "You're shaving!!!" (says monitor)

Supervisors in the residence shared and encouraged the monitors' sentiments; self-sufficiency and independent decision-making were valued and, thus, routinely encouraged.

> Observation: *Mrs. Segal heads toward the elevator.*
> RESIDENT NURSE MILLER: (to the observer) She's a real resident. She came in here herself. She wasn't sick. She takes her own meds. She's really on the go. . . . We encourage decision-making over here. "What do you want? What do you want to wear . . . to do?" They don't do that over there. (intermediate unit)

In the context of our concerns about role relationships, the phrase "she is a real resident" is particularly interesting. Ms. Miller is defining the features of the normative role by example, and the emphasis is on autonomy and activity.

Despite physical and cognitive screening and a mobility criterion, quite a few residents exhibited both physical and mental deterioration. This did not go unrecognized by the monitors.

> RESIDENT MONITOR BLACK: . . . technically they are supposed to be self-sufficient. They are free to come and go, to make their own doctor appointments. But not too many of them can. If they get a doctor's office that [is playing a] recording, they're (residents) saying, "I don't understand." And then we intercede for them. . . . So they're not as independent or self-sufficient as we'd like them to be. . . . Yea, we are seeing more of the residents become patients if only because we're dealing with a longer period of time. You know, they are with us a longer period and it's just a degenerative thing.
> OBSERVER: Are they pretty resistant to being sent over there? (reference to intermediate care)
> MS. BLACK: Normally when they are in declining health, they have no choice. When they're mobile and ambulatory and active they want nothing to do with the skilled side because to them that means sickness and death and separation.

In some cases the impairments created only minimal extra work for residential staff and, in these cases, an approach that maximized residents' autonomy and protected their self-esteem without sacrificing physical well-being was generally adopted.

> RESIDENT MONITOR BLACK: . . . Mrs. Miller goes and falls asleep, and wakes up and thinks it's breakfast time when it might be supper time or lunch, you know? My philosophy is that they aren't patients. They are free to come and go, as long they are not hurting themselves, or endangering themselves, or disturbing their fellow residents or hurting them. I kinda let them go. If I know they are off the unit I'll kinda spot-check them. I'll keep an eye on them. But I don't try to confine them because I feel that only frustrates them more. So I give them some freedom as long as they're not in pain and hurting themselves, or causing pain or harm to anybody else. So, if a nurse calls and says, "Hey, I saw Elizabeth Miller down in the lobby," I say, "Thanks, I'll go down and get her."

The more extensive impairment of other residents required a considerable amount of extra work by the monitors.

> Resident Monitor Olsen: Mary has become incontinent about urine. She wears Depends. She is so confused that she does not know how to put the Depends on, and she's been in them for months and months and months. I have gone in I can't tell you how many times to find the Depend fastened around the small of her back. Now the dirty band is on her back, and she thinks she's ready to start the day. She sleeps in the nude with newspapers . . . wrapped up in different dresses and housecoats . . . .

Considering the staffing in the residential areas (one resident monitor per fifteen residents), common sense suggests that encouraging residents to be independent and self-sufficient would help the units to run smoothly. The logical extension of that approach would dictate the removal of residents no longer able to function for the most part on their own. However, we found that resident monitors frequently compensated for failing physical and cognitive functioning of residents in order that those individuals could remain on the residential units. The willingness of staff to pick up the slack for failing residents appears to be a function both of the unit's basic philosophy and the close relationships between many residential staff and residents.

> Observer: It sounds like you know these people pretty well.
> Resident Monitor Black: Yea, I love them. I really do. I just see them as human beings.
> Resident Monitor Johnson: . . . we're . . . supposed to be able to maintain a relationship between the family and them (residents). We're supposed to keep in contact with the family, the members of the family, the friends, you know. We are their family. We take them in and we surround them. Do you understand what I'm saying?
> Observer: Yes.
> Ms. Olson: That's our job.

This approach, however, was conditional in that it did not extend to residents whom the monitors thought had been mistakenly admitted to the residential area. As we saw in the previous chapter, staff had rather little tolerance for those who did not show sufficient enthusiasm for their own independence.

This exception notwithstanding, it seems that staff-resident relationships built on the conceptualization of residents as unique individuals helps to buffer the impact of later physical and cognitive deterioration. We saw many examples in which monitors inconvenienced themselves in order to help such residents remain in independent living. Similar relationships, however, failed to develop between monitors and residents impaired at the time of admission. Residential staff comments indicated their conceptualization of these individuals as patients and their preference for their transfer to intermediate or skilled care. One obvious implication is that the initial staff conceptualization of an individual's role (as patient or "unique individual") dictates not only the parameters of that individual's sanctioned behaviors within the specified setting, but the responses of others to those behaviors.

Conclusion

The differences in the model of staff and resident roles between the nursing home and the residence seems to explain many of the differences between the two settings. In the residence sustaining autonomous functioning, not health care, seemed the dominant value among line staff. Monitors, rather than viewing themselves as medical personnel, saw their role as helping the residents live their lives (as the residents defined them). These differences seem to us to be built into the fact that the nursing home was organized around a medical model, while the residential setting was seen as providing a place where residents could live autonomously. Whatever the blessings of a medical model for the elderly in long-term care, promoting independence is not one of them.

6

Restrictions

In the previous two chapters, we looked at the nature of the value structures and role relationships in the intermediate and skilled care and residence settings. Caregiver-patient relationships seem to be derivative of the traditional physician-patient relationship, while staff-resident relationships are more reminiscent of those seen between the elderly and supportive family members. These findings have important consequences for the ideals of autonomy.

This chapter, however, is concerned with what might be called "liberty issues," ie, the pattern of restrictions imposed on patients so that the institution can function efficiently and achieve its goals. In particular, staff believe that they need to restrict patients and their actions in order to protect their safety and keep them in good medical condition. Such restrictions are a central feature of institutional life in nursing homes and are thus of central importance to our task.

Before we begin a review of the types of restrictions that existed for patients and residents, it will be helpful to discuss briefly two contrasting approaches to liberty. In the traditional liberal theory of autonomy, perhaps best elaborated by John Stuart Mill (1955), restrictions are clearly antithetical to autonomy. Typically, a person's ability to choose for herself the kind of life she wants to live decreases as the number of restrictions or "closed options" increases.[1] Thus, for Mill, the only justification for restricting the liberty of one human being is that it interferes with the rights of others. A person's freedom and, to a lesser degree, her autonomy, are undercut precisely to the degree that behavior is restricted (Mill 1955).

A somewhat different position can be found in the work of the classic social theorist Emile Durkheim. In his study of suicide, Durkheim pointed out that the absence of external guidance leads to a loss of orientation and direction that he called "anomie" (Durkheim 1951). In short, people cannot autonomously direct their lives in a social vacuum, but rely on the social institutions and groups in which they live to structure choices and provide direction. Somewhat less well known is Durkheim's analysis of "fatalism," which suggests that suicides also occur frequently in contexts in which the agent perceives no choices whatsoever.

For our purposes it does not matter whether or not Durkheim was correct about the origins of suicide. What matters is his basic view regarding the role of restrictions in social life and their impact on a person's ability to live autonomously. For Durkheim there can be no social life without normatively based restrictions. Such norms guide the choices we make, giving us a sense of direction with which to orient our actions. It is only within such normative regulation that we can expect to see autonomous activity. What one would hope to find in a long-term care setting, from a Durkheimian perspective, is that the restrictions are rationally related to the legitimate institutional goals and that a substantial effort has been made to individualize the restrictions.

It is important to note that neither Mill nor Durkheim provides any direction on one of the fundamental problems that arises in nursing homes, namely formulating restrictions for a group of individuals with varying abilities to act autonomously. While Durkheim does not assume that rational individuals pursue enlightened self-interest, he does assume the ability to orient one's behavior vis-a-vis societal values. What happens when that capacity is not there is no more clear in Durkheim's writings than in those of classical liberal theorists.[2]

Institutional restrictions played a significant role in a variety of different decisions: who would be admitted; who would be discharged or transferred to another facility or among various in-house units; what forms of treatment would be provided; what behaviors would be tolerated under what circumstances; and how, where, and with whom patients would spend their waking hours. In short, institutional restrictions dealt with nearly every facet of patients and residents' lives. We cannot review all of these restrictions here, but we will focus on their major dimensions and how they were carried out in the nursing home settings.

Some of the restrictions (eg, admission and discharge, insurance-reimbursed treatments,) were partly a result of rules generated outside the institution and were merely enforced or not enforced by the facility staff. The rest were developed by the facility staff to advance their goals. These restrictions took a variety of forms. First, every institution has a fairly extensive set of institutional policies. These formal restrictions largely reflect the goals and values of the upper staff. For these rules to have an effect on patient care, however, lower staff must enforce them. Informal restrictions were also important in regulating patient and resident behavior. Staff, in the course of their day-to-day work, developed a set of rules to restrict and punish selected patient behavior. These rules were enforced within the facility with a surprising degree of consistency, using both subtle forms of interpersonal persuasion and physical force to assure compliance.

In order to examine the nature of these restrictions we reviewed all of the coded instances of staff "proscriptions" and "prescriptions" (Merton 1949) for patient behavior. After extensive review, three categories of restrictions emerged:

1. Restrictions focused on preserving the body.
2. Restrictions that complied with regulatory and in-house policies, in particular policies that affected reimbursement.
3. Maintenance of institutional routines.

Preserving the Body

Preserving the Body in the Nursing Home

We noted previously that physical care was high on the list of values of staff, families, and patients. Indeed, physical care was probably the dominant value, reflecting the medical model on which the nursing home functioned. A significant number of the restrictions that we observed were related directly to the perceived need to maintain patients' physical integrity. Restrictions that were designed to safeguard the physical integrity of patients took a variety of forms including physical restraints, restrictions to prevent inter-patient violence, and a variety of restrictions on treatment and discharge.

Physical Restraints. Both the most pervasive and the most invasive form of patient management was the use of physical restraints. We will discuss the use of restraints in detail in Chapter 10, but an overview is necessary here.

Restraints were common on both the intermediate and skilled/intermediate units, and were used most often with cognitively impaired individuals. The majority of intermediate unit patients, as well as a large number of skilled/intermediate patients were restrained on a regular basis. While the numbers of those restrained varied from week to week, it was always high. On one randomly chosen day on the intermediate care unit, 12% were restrained in their beds, 27% in geri-chairs, and 49% in wheelchairs. Only 12% were unrestrained. The following are routine observations from our notes:

> Observation: *Mr. McLaughlin is drooling a lot. He's tied in a wheelchair and is wearing a rubber bib. He slowly rolls himself forward and backward. His wife sits in a chair and watches.*
> Observation: *Mrs. Linley (aide) rolls Hilda Kramer down the hallway and back to the lounge. Hilda is tied in the geri-chair and is wearing a bib.*

The impact of physical restraint on a patient's liberty is largely a function of the type of restraint used. Patients' mobility and, therefore, their social lives and activities were affected to differing degrees by the different forms of restraints. The three most common mechanisms for restraining patients were wheelchairs, geri-chairs, and bed restraints. Patients restrained in wheelchairs, but with the strength to wheel themselves, were relatively free to determine where and with whom they would spend their days. Patients relegated to geri-chairs were mobile only if staff were willing to move them. However, since geri-chairs were generally placed in the lounge area or hallway, these patients were still able to communicate with most other patients. Those patients restrained in bed were the most severely affected. They lacked both mobility and the opportunity to interact with any individuals who did not explicitly come to see them.

However, such a characterization of the use of restraints must be qualified somewhat by the realization that not all patients are alike in their capability to interact with others. Thus, most patients who were restrained in bed were largely incapable of interacting with others. On the other hand, less impaired and more active (the noisiest and most demanding) patients were generally restrained in geri-chairs. This does not mean that restraints did not adversely affect patients' freedom; however the use of restraints further limited patients who were already limited by their mental and physical disabilities.[3]

Patient Conflicts. In an effort to promote patient safety, staff developed a series of restrictions to prevent inter-patient aggression. The following example is a typical account of staff response to such aggression.

> US–01: Mary Camden . . . she's a real character. You want to see a classic . . . it's probably too late now because Elizabeth's so sick . . .

> a classic case of sibling rivalry. We had to banish her for a while because one day the staff caught her hitting Elizabeth. "Betta (US–01 repeats Mary's use of an ethnic variation of Elizabeth's first name) "Betta, you're just too lazy to walk! Now you just get out of that chair and walk! Wap!" (US–01 imitates Mary hitting Elizabeth)
>
> OBSERVER: Ooh.
>
> US–01: Can you believe that? So Mary was banished for awhile. Now Mary has her limits.
>
> OBSERVER: What are they?
>
> US–01: She knows that she can't stay a long time, and staff keeps a really close watch on her. . . .

In this case, the visitation restrictions served the obvious function of preventing the resident from injuring her sister and may have served as a punishment for the previous aggression. The staff supervision was also symbolic of their concern for patients' physical well-being.

In making these decisions, the upper staff tried to balance their concern for Elizabeth's physical health with Mary's right to do what she wanted. They did not, for example, completely prevent Mary from interacting with her sister. However, the predominance of the concern for protecting physical well-being is reflected in staff's failure to try other approaches. Talking with Mary about not injuring her sister may have left Elizabeth's safety at higher risk but would have been more consistent with Mary's autonomy. Strict restrictions on Mary and Elizabeth's interactions limited one of their few remaining long-standing relationships.

However, inter-patient aggression was not always so tightly restricted. In one series of instances staff showed considerable ambivalence about how much they should restrict conflict between a married couple. Mild aggression between Mr. and Mrs. Friedman was often the final observed link in a chain of negative interactions between the two patients. Sarah, an aphasic stroke patient, would frequently try to communicate with her husband and, failing in these attempts, would begin crying and screaming. Bernard would reciprocate by first yelling, and then—if Sarah continued to yell—by leaving the area, which usually further upset his wife. Without intervention by staff or family, this series of interactions would, at times, end in mild aggression (eg, Mr. Friedman would grab his wife's arm to prevent her from moving away from him, or Mrs. Friedman would slap at her husband or grab at his clothing).

Staff felt they had reason to worry that these fights would result in more serious consequences. Sarah had suffered various injuries (eg, broken arm, broken finger) that did not clearly result from a fall or other mishap. Upper staff told us that they tried to suggest to the patients' daughter that her mother's injuries might have been the result of aggression by her father; the daughter, however, did not consider this possible. On the other hand, sometimes it appeared that Mrs. Friedman was actually the aggressor.

> MS. DAVIS (aide): (rolling her eyes) . . . You should see her. (referring to Mrs. Friedman) She beats him up. (referring to Mr. Friedman)
> OBSERVER: Really?
> MS. DAVIS: Yeah. And you better watch or she'll beat on you, too. You know, when he was here before . . . when he used to visit her, every once in a while we would find him on the floor in her room. And you know what? She was tripping him. She would just stick out her foot in front of him. One day we saw her do it.

However, unlike the case of the two sisters, staff did not systematically attempt to separate Mr. and Mrs. Friedman. Instead, the problem was managed on an incident-by-incident basis.

> Observation: *[Bernard and Sarah Friedman are] sitting in wheelchairs by the elevator. The woman, Sarah, is crying loudly. She is grasping at the front of . . . [Bernard's] shirt.*
> MRS. BROSKY (aide): Don't.
> Observation: *Mrs. Brosky rolls Bernard away from Sarah. She rolls him to a position in front of the television set. Sarah cries louder.*
> MRS. BROSKY: (to her) He's going to watch some TV. Do you want to watch, too?
> SARAH: Mama. (sobbing)

Several factors may account for the difference between the response to Mr. and Mrs. Friedman, on one hand, and Mary and Elizabeth on the other. First, the context in which the injuries to Sarah occurred is unclear, while staff clearly witnessed Mary's assaults on her sister. Moreover, the fact that both Sarah and Bernard were confined to wheelchairs may have given the staff a sense of control over the conflict that they did not have with Mary, who could get around independently. Moreover, Bernard and Sarah were living on the same unit and this made it relatively more difficult to limit their contact.

It is also important to note that Elizabeth's husband, also an impaired patient, was living on the same unit with his wife, while Mr. and Mrs. Friedman were not related to any other patients or residents. Therefore, restricting Mary from visiting her sister did not completely deprive Elizabeth of familial support, while the same type of intervention (eg, relocating either Bernard or Sarah) would have severely restricted their interactions. Whatever the specifics of the case, it seems clear that staff took potential injuries to one patient by another seriously enough to put substantial restrictions on the interactions between patients but not seriously enough to severely restrict the husband-wife relationship. While one might quarrel with the particular resolution, it seems that the staff were making distinctions between the two cases that reflected their assessment of conflicting values.

Decisions Regarding Treatment and Discharge. So far we have focused on the informal restrictions lower staff have used in their routine management of patients. We have suggested that patient safety and physical health norms seem to orient staff behavior in such a way that substantial restrictions on patients' behaviors were seen as appropriate.

Decisions about treatment and discharge, however, were made largely by upper staff who not only expressed different values but also seemed less inclined to restrict patients' behavior. One situation in which upper staff members frequently supported a patient's decision, rather than focusing exclusively on her physical health, concerned the right to die. Although the following incident involves only one upper staff member, other upper staff repeatedly expressed the same support for a patient's right to refuse life-sustaining treatment.

> US–03: We had another lady, Helen. She was in her nineties. Verbally had said for the past three years to her family, "Please let me die." She had lived at home, had almost deliberately cut and tapered her food off to just liquids. She wanted to die. She had no reason to live anymore. But they (family) were determined to find an excuse to get her into a hospital. And I'll be doggoned if they didn't. She had passed out or something, and they had her admitted. Worked her up over there (hospital). And then she came here. She begged and screamed and hollered. Whipped out tubes . . . I bet in a month we put in . . .
> OBSERVER: A patient can't refuse to have tubes put in?
> US–03: Sure, they can.
> OBSERVER: But they're put in anyway?
> US–03: Yes.
> OBSERVER: Who makes the decision about whether a tube is put in?
> US–03: Usually the family.
> OBSERVER: Did she have a guardian?

US–03: No, she was fully competent. But to prove this . . . I felt really strongly about allowing this woman her right to die. But I can't barge in and tell a practicing RN, who has her own ethical values and morals, and who knew it was a physician's order . . . She'd say, "There's an order there. I have to put it back in. You know she'll die if she doesn't have that." Her physician here was Dr. X, who feels very, very strongly about keeping . . . I shouldn't say keeping people alive. He's not that . . . but with naso-gastric tubes . . . he's like really adamant about you keeping those in. So he felt that it should be kept in.

OBSERVER: Did he put it in?

US–03: No, the nursing staff always put it in because she'd whip them out so frequently.

OBSERVER: That figures. But he wrote the order?

US–03: That's correct. And we'd call him, and he'd say, "Put another one back in."

OBSERVER: How did her family feel about this?

US–03: OK. That was the other sensitive issue. She had 2 sons and a daughter. One son was on our side and did not want it put back in. The other son and daughter wanted everything done to keep mother alive. So then we invited all of them to a patient care conference. One of them showed up and he was able to verbalize. "Look, I know that mother wants to die." He was the one who was very supportive of us. . . . We decided to get Dr. Y to come in for a competency consult.

OBSERVER: He's the . . . ?

US–03: Y's the psychiatrist. So we finally got the family to agree to a psych consult. . . . He came and said that she was not incompetent, but that she had a right to say that she was ready to die and she should be able to say it. With that in mind, the family agreed to leave the tube out. I don't know why. I don't know why even today, but she started to eat. . . . She ate enough that she finally did go home.

It should be clear that the placing or removing of restrictions on this patient was not simply a matter of the staff member's choice or values. While disinclined to restrict this patient's right to die, US–03 clearly had a complex political game to play in order to free the patient from the institutionalized bias to prolong life. Only when she was supported by the psychiatrist could she mobilize the support necessary to override the restrictions designed to protect the patient's health.

The complexities of deciding when to protect patients' bodily well-being versus allowing patients to do as they choose is well illustrated in the following case. It involves the even more complicated problem of integrating physician, guardian, and patient preferences. The patient, admitted to the facility for rehabilitation following a hip fracture, wanted to go home. Based in part on the nature of the accident (the patient fell after tripping over a rug in her home), the patient's assigned physician and her guardians felt that the patient's return to her pre-accident lifestyle would place her at risk for another accident. They therefore requested that she modify her living arrangements, including limiting her living space to the first floor of her home, using personal care aides in the home during the day, and putting her dog in the basement at night, to minimize the possibility of another fall. To this end, the guardians recruited an upper staff member to negotiate terms, a process that extended over much of the six-month data collection period.

> Observation: *The staff member and patient are sitting in the patient's room.*
> US–02: We don't want you to fall down and have to come back to us. If you walk in the door, fine. If not, well. . . . Perhaps some of what you have to do will be to compromise.
> Observation: *US–02 shakes the walker.*
> US–02: You know, we'll have to order you one of your own.
> MRS. BAKER: Yes, this is wonderful.
> US–02: Yes. You'll need one upstairs and downstairs.
> MRS. BAKER: Yes, that could work well.
> US–02: OK. We don't want to see you fall again.
> MRS. BAKER: No.
> US–02: And you might need some help with other things. Like bathing.
> MRS. BAKER: No, I don't bathe. I just take sponge baths.
> US–02: But . . .
> MRS. BAKER: (interrupts) I've taken sponge baths since my husband died.
> US–02: What about a shower?
> MRS. BAKER: Those shower things just aren't for me.
> US–02: OK. Well, to close—you're going to think about what we've said? There are some things you might want to do. And there are some things we'll need to do before you leave.
> MRS. BAKER: Well, you know, I just don't want to keep Brandy (her dog) out at night.
> US–02: Well, you would just have to keep her down at night.
> MRS. BAKER: Well, she might not be happy that way.

US–02: I don't know if her happiness is the bottom line here, honey.
Observation: *US–02 reaches out and pats the patient on her knee. Then she leaves the room and goes down toward the staff area to answer a page. As she goes down the hall, she speaks to me.*
US–02: This is what I mean by compromise. Having the dog in the cellar is one way of helping to prevent another fall. . . .

Mrs. Baker, however, was an intensely private person who had not adjusted well to the lack of privacy inherent in institutional living or to separation from her pet. Throughout the data collection period, she reiterated her desire for discharge and to return to her previous lifestyle. For example:

MRS. BAKER: There are two beds in here and things get crowded, too. Some of my family [reference is to guardians, whom, although not close relatives, the patient refers to as family] wants me to live here.
OBSERVER: Is that what you want?
MRS. BAKER: No. There are too many things crowding into my desires. If I just had one member of my [immediate] family alive, how happy I would be. But, I'll adjust I guess. And I won't expect everything to be perfect. It never was that way. I never had that. All of my life. And I've always had dogs. . . . Yes. I'm not a bit scared at night. You know, prowlers and burglars and such with a dog. (pause) Brandy. That's her name.
OBSERVER: I bet she has missed you.
MRS. BAKER: Yea, and I've missed her, too.

While US–03 was aware of the patient's feelings, an impromptu tour of Mrs. Baker's house reinforced the concern for her physical well-being.

US–03: We've (staff) had many, many conferences together as to what to do for Gertrude Baker. . . . Always lived by herself. She was a relative recluse. She had been married. She's a widow. She has no children. She has some neighbors that were supportive friends. And she had her dog at home. She literally lived at home by herself for many, many years. [When she got here] all she wanted was to go home. [A] good friend of Gertrude's knew a lot about her. She took (staff) to her house to go up and see what it was like. It was literally like a packrat house. . . . She had stuff everywhere, piled high to the sky. Saved everything. There were scatter rugs everywhere. She had sweaters laying around that had been patched. She had chairs . . . I mean the place was filled with gorgeous antique furniture. She had a

> huge baby grand piano. She had bookcases that had gold leaf bound books everywhere. The house was just a gold mine for antiques. But the chairs, some of the chairs had holes in them in the seat. It was like she probably existed in that room . . . very, very happily. But to us, it looked like "My God, you can kill yourself here." And now going back after a fractured hip, with scatter rugs around and her little dog in there, we didn't think it was really safe. . . .

Although US–02 was initially supportive of trying to modify the patient's living situation before releasing her, she slowly grew less enthusiastic as an increasingly clear conflict emerged between the patient's wishes and the guardians' desires to restrict her to the nursing home. In the latter stages of negotiation, US–02 indicated her belief that concern for the patient's well-being was being used to disguise a desire to keep the patient in the nursing facility.

> Observation: *Mrs. Baker eventually agrees (albeit reluctantly) to consider the residence as an alternative to intermediate care in the event that she could not return home.*
> US–02: Gertrude is in tears because she misses her dog and she wants to go home. The doctor has told her that he wants her to walk more and to stay here for another three months. She's decided that she wants to go back and see the residence area again.
> OBSERVER: OK.
> US–02: I think the [guardians are] wearing her down by attrition. . . . They're just stringing her out because they don't want her to go back home.

As negotiation continued, US–02 began to notice negative effects on the patient resulting from continued institutionalization.

> US–02: Mrs. Baker has gotten lost in the shuffle. I have seen her caregivers and they're going to wait until the doctor's appointment. I don't know what Gertrude's feelings are right now. I'm worried that Gertrude is getting very institutionalized, to be honest with you. Which is what the caregivers wanted to happen.
> OBSERVER: They don't want her back?
> US–02: No. They don't want her in that house and have to worry about her. Mrs. Baker, to me, is very much in a borderline situation. We took Gertrude up to the residence once. She didn't like it. She still wanted to go home.

OBSERVER: I'm curious. How do you define becoming institutionalized?
US–02: Becoming more passive, not interacting, or just giving in to the system. Gertrude, to me, is in a gray zone. If she wants to go home, that would give her some quality of life.

These decisions about what sorts of restrictions to place on patients—both regarding the refusal of life-sustaining treatment and the right to choose one's living situation—are not simple one-factor decisions. Upper staff must consider both their strong commitment to the patient's physical well-being and their commitment to protecting the patient's ability to choose for herself. When these values conflict, however, a variety of factors conspire to restrict patient autonomy and err on the side of protecting the patient's physical well-being. The patient's family are often more concerned with the patient's health than their ability to choose, particularly when they do not agree with the patient's choice. The cases described above also point out the ways in which the value of physical well-being was integrated into the institutional structure of the nursing home. Finally, nursing homes have a legal obligation to insure the well-being of their clients and this is usually interpretated as an obligation to promote their physical health. Given the potential legal and regulatory problems that may result from failure to adequately care for the physical condition of the patients, such personal and institutional values are not easily changed.

Preserving the Body in the Residence

From what we have previously said about the residence, one would not expect to find restrictions imposed for residents' physical well-being without their consent. It was, therefore, somewhat surprising to find that residents capable of meeting the physical demands of residential living, but with suspect cognitive function, were bound by some of the same restrictions as the physically and mentally impaired patients in the intermediate care facility. Restrictions were justified as preventing physical harm.

For example, despite the staff's belief that Mrs. Zabotnik might be capable of self-medication, and without formal assessment of cognitive function or a documented history of medication mismanagement, she was largely prevented from managing her own medications.[4]

N–02: . . . the only thing Mrs. Zabotnik keeps is nitroglycerin . . . little tablets for under her tongue for angina.
OBSERVER: And she keeps those?

> N–02: Yes, she's allowed to have so many at a time. (pause) If she had them all I think she would abuse that.
> OBSERVER: Has she abused it in the past?
> N–02: I think she has. I can't say that I've actually seen her do it, but sometimes she thinks they're something else . . . .
> OBSERVER: Can she get her prescriptions filled on her own?
> UPPER STAFF: No, she's not able to. And she knows that.

This particular restriction was apparently quite upsetting to the resident, a retired registered nurse.

> N–02: [Elaine] was a registered nurse. "I am a nurse and I used to give medicine to other people. Who do you think you are to give me my medicine?" You know? . . . And it's tough for her to accept me making sure she gets medicine.

Restrictions for the purpose of protecting the physical well-being of cognitively impaired patients are relatively easy to justify. Even J. S. Mill restricted his notions of liberty to adults of sound mind. For many, if not most of these individuals, the ability to initiate goal-oriented activity is quite limited and, thus, the autonomy lost is more limited. Thus, safety-related restrictions are easier to justify in the intermediate care facility, particularly for the more demented patients.[5]

The application of such restrictions to less impaired individuals, however, poses a greater conflict with patient or resident self-determination. Consider the following example: a reasonably healthy, cognitively intact resident with no history of injury related to the specific restriction was forbidden to help a patient leave the dining area.

> MRS. BLACK (resident monitor): He (John Taylor) likes to help. He loves to help and volunteer help. He began to push a patient in a wheelchair. Now this is a no-no policy to begin with. . . . After witnessing the little (dizziness) spell he had, I didn't want him pushing 125 pounds in a chair. So I got up from the table and I said, "Mr. Taylor, I'll do that." He said, "That's OK. I'm going down the elevator." I said, "No thanks, I'll do that." I really had to insist.

The resident monitor was clearly trying to be helpful. She was going beyond the call of duty since resident monitors are not responsible for patients, and moving this patient resulted in some inconvenience. However, the resident was perfectly capable of making his own judgements.

This resident monitor was, like her colleagues in the intermediate and skilled care settings, willing to restrict her charges' liberty to ensure their physical well-being.

Unfortunately, our data concerning restrictions justified on the basis of safety or well-being in the residential care facility is fairly limited. Moreover, comparisons between restrictions for the mobile residents and the largely immobile intermediate care patients are difficult. Still, it is our impression that the massive difference in autonomy between the two settings is not primarily due to differences in the willingness of staff to restrict patients or residents because of concerns regarding their physical well-being.

Compliance with Fiscal Policies

Not all restrictions imposed on the patients and residents were focused on concern for health or safety. Nursing homes, like most other institutions in our society, are regulated by a variety of governmental and quasi-governmental agencies and have their own in-house policies based on a variety of rationales. However, many restrictions were justified directly on the basis of regulatory and in-house policies.

Regulations concerning the financing of nursing homes have played an important role in modifying patient care, albeit indirectly. This is particularly true in determining where, for what, and for how long patients and residents would reside. Questions concerning admission, treatment for patients, and discharge were regularly discussed at the weekly discharge and planning meetings that were attended by the executive director, social worker, clinical specialist, nursing supervisor, physical and occupational therapists, and the admissions coordinator.

A picture of these meetings can be gained from a discussion of the possibility of releasing a patient with limited financial resources to home care.

> NURSING SUPERVISOR: OK. This is Bessie Stephens. She's 80 years old. She's not doing super in her work.
> OCCUPATIONAL THERAPIST: She's not going anywhere.
> PHYSICAL THERAPIST: Her progress is very slow. She's taking two to three shuffling steps now in the parallel bars.
> OCCUPATIONAL THERAPIST: She's at least learned to assist herself some with transfers. She used to be a full person, but now she's able to try to shift her weight to a good leg and pivot. I'm not sure how good that is for her ankle though. Cracking noises everywhere. She must have

had home care of some kind to make it at home and survive the way she was.

ADMISSIONS COORDINATOR: When she was home she had someone from the Area Association on Aging coming in?

PHYSICAL THERAPIST: Yeah.

SOCIAL WORKER: How much does she have in PT? (reference to amount of reimbursable physical therapy left)

PHYSICAL THERAPIST: She's gonna have to start making progress to continue to get PT.

SOCIAL WORKER: She may not get to her apartment. She wants to, but she's also afraid to. She's afraid of falling again, but she sees the alternative as not too great.

ADMISSIONS COORDINATOR: She's starting to look like long-term care.

OCCUPATIONAL THERAPIST: (county facility)?

SOCIAL WORKER: Probably so.

OCCUPATIONAL THERAPIST: She's such a nice lady. Every bone cracked so badly.

PHYSICAL THERAPIST: And when she doesn't get PT anymore, she'll begin to stiffen.

SOCIAL WORKER: The shame is that she's so mentally alert.

While the staff members appeared to support her goal to return home, they saw it as unrealistic based on her inability to achieve the required progress in physical therapy. The staff seem to take rehabilitation progress, remaining reimbursement, and the minimum requirements for independent living into consideration when determining whether or not discharge is "possible." Patient preferences play a significant role in this decision-making process only when the patient's desires are seen as "realistic" in the context of both institutional and governmental fiscal policies.

A similar pattern occurred in the following case:

NURSING SUPERVISOR: Mr. Owen is 77-year-old man with peptic ulcer disease, a hip replacement, diabetes mellitus, and is receiving medication. He has a central line in and is getting Vancomycin, which is to be changed to Keflex in a few days.

SOCIAL WORKER: Is that still by IV? (ie, will Medicare coverage continue?)

NURSING SUPERVISOR: THAT'S STILL IV. . . .

OBSERVATION: *Clinical specialist looks at occupational therapist and physical therapist.*

PHYSICAL THERAPIST: It's slow. Very slow.

OBSERVATION: *Occupational Therapist and Physical Therapist begin to describe particulars of rehabilitation. All begin to discuss possible changes in lifestyle such as a change to an apartment without steps, putting the bed on the first floor, the wife decreasing her outside activities and her expectations for her husband.*
NURSING SUPERVISOR: Then as soon as the IV comes out, that's it. (reference to end of Medicare coverage)
OBSERVATION: *All continue to try to figure out his medical situation to see how long his insurance will continue.*
NURSING SUPERVISOR: Does he have more rehab time?
PHYSICAL THERAPIST: He's rehab'ed out.
SOCIAL WORKER: He'll have to have an attendant at home, or she'll have to help a lot more, or he'll have to go to a personal care home. He needs assistance. She's not ready for this. She'll bring him back, because she's not ready. I hope she doesn't verbally abuse him. This is an accident waiting to happen.
NURSING SUPERVISOR: We can't protect the world.
SOCIAL WORKER: I don't think she can handle him.

Here, as elsewhere, when the staff are discussing a patient whose insurance reimbursement will be discontinued, the assumption is that issues about financing are essentially fixed whether her rehabilitation goals are met or not. In other words, the reimbursement structure is perceived as an external constraint. The staff do not see themselves as responsible for these restrictions on patient care. They are "regrettable but something we can do nothing about." Consequently, there is no option of remaining at the facility for further treatment unless the patient (or the legal guardian) can assume financial responsibility for continuing care.

Despite the "necessity" of discharge, it was apparent that various staff members did not feel that the patient described above would be able to manage at home without considerable assistance. Several features of the patient's home environment further constrained his choices:

Note: *From a later discussion.*
US–02: You know Mr. Owen on the fifth floor?
OBSERVER: He has the wife with the . . . ah . . . active lifestyle who doesn't want him to come home?
US–02: Yeah. I think we can get him into personal care. . . . I'm really concerned about Mr. Owen's safety because it's been discovered that the wife has a drinking problem.
OBSERVER: Do you suspect that she abused him?

> US–02: One older son says that she does things to him. . . . So after I find out whether it is feasible, I'll put him, his son, and his wife in a van and take a little trip down to this personal care home . . . .

In this case the combination of poor social support and the policy dictating the amount of reimbursable rehabilitation reduced the patient's options and put him at high risk for receiving inferior care. US–02 attempted to circumvent this possibility by encouraging the patient and his family to consider transfer to a personal care facility instead of discharging him home. The patient's preferences in this decision appeared to play at best a minor role in the decision-making process.

While in most instances the staff treated reimbursement and other policy criteria as though they were external immutable constraints on their treatment and disposition choices, this was not always so:

> Note: (*From an interview with an upper staff member.*) *Once the tape recorder was turned off, she freely admitted that they will sometimes stop a patient from walking 100 feet, regardless of whether the patient can walk that distance, if the length of that walk itself would necessitate termination of the patient's physical therapy reimbursement while other needs remain to be met.*

It is interesting to note that these exceptions were made when the staff felt that the patient needed further care, rather than when the patient requested further care. These exceptions once again point out the primacy of "medical well-being" in the staff's decision-making process.

Although for the most part governmental policies controlled length and type of coverage, in-house policies regarding reimbursement were most important in setting admissions criteria. In cases where applicants held a variety of coverages (eg, Medicare, private insurance, self-pay), the type of coverage appeared to take a back seat to the attempt by administrators to keep the beds filled (openings were filled from the top of the waiting list without reference to method of payment). The role of institutional policies regarding admission and their impact on patient care will be explored in more detail later.

We noted earlier that there were no strong differences between the residence and skilled/intermediate care concerning how restrictive the settings were in their protection of physical health and safety. However, there were quite striking differences in the degree to which governmental fiscal policies restricted resident choices for the simple reason that there was no third-party reimbursement for the residential side. Since there was no third-party reimbursement, insurance regulation could not restrict resident choices. Only the lack of private financial resources to pay for room and board restricted residents' choices about entering or leaving the residence.[6]

Maintenance of Institutional Routines

Intermediate/Skilled Care

While fiscal restrictions and concerns for health and safety provide a consistent background against which particular patients' choices and activities are constrained, there is another group of restrictions that are at least as subversive of patient autonomy. These restrictions are undertaken in the interests of intra-institutional order and efficiency.

Nursing facilities, like all other organizations, have procedures and routines for accomplishing their tasks. Since these tasks involve the care and maintenance of patients, any routine for accomplishing those tasks is likely to have an impact on patients' abilities to do what they want, when they want. Specifically, institutional procedures often dictate where, when, and how patients spent their waking hours. These sorts of restrictions occur across a variety of contexts and staff levels, and lead to widespread interference with patient and resident autonomy. While these restrictions are based on a variety of staff goals, the fundamental aim is to maximize the efficient use of staff time.

These restrictions were designed primarily for the more physically and mentally impaired patients whose management was more difficult and time consuming. In many cases, these restrictions can be viewed as structuring the environment of patients who were unable to provide their own structure. In most of these situations, patients were given no options but to comply with the staff-imposed routines.

> Observation: *I was walking a quite impaired patient down to the dining room.*
> OBSERVER: Where do you want to go?
> MRS. KAZMERIC: I don't know.
> Observation: *An aide walks up to us.*
> AIDE: Monica sits over here.
> Observation: *The aide takes Mrs. Kazmeric over to her seat, where she sits down.*

This interaction reflects a basic fact about nursing homes. Chronically understaffed and faced with patients who are unable to make decisions for themselves or whose choices make management difficult, such facilities develop ways to improve efficiency. A common response is to make a large number of rules about what patients should do—in other words to routinize care. In this case, patients who ate in the dining room were given assigned seats that they were not to change by themselves. If a patient wanted to change seats she had to request such a change from staff.

Line staff routinely appealed to these restrictions to help them carry out their everyday tasks:

> Observation: *Mrs. Kazmeric walks down from the dining hall (with an aide). She really looks out of it.*
> AIDE: Now you wait right here for your bus.
> Observation: *It is not clear to me what she (aide) is talking about. The aide walks back down the hallway toward the dining room. Mrs. Kazmeric waits for about thirty seconds, then follows the aide. . . . The elevator comes and another patient gets on. As she does, the aide brings Mrs. Kazmeric back down the hallway. This time she parks her on the couch.*
> AIDE: (emphatically) You wait for the elevator here!
> Observation: *The aide heads back up the hallway toward the dining room.*

Every setting had a routine set of rules designed to simplify staff tasks by allowing all patients to be treated as more or less identical problems to be managed.

> Observation: *About three-quarters of the way through the meal Mrs. Carl attempted to leave the dining room. She began to roll her wheelchair toward the door. She was confronted by the dining room monitor. She was told in no uncertain terms that she "knew the rules" and that she knew she could not leave the room until everyone was done. Mrs. Carl protested that she was finished with her meal, and should be allowed to go back upstairs. The monitor blocked her way.*

The notion that all patients should be treated as identically was, however, more than just an instrumentally useful rule; it became a fundamental normative expectation among line staff. Thus, regardless of their mental or physical capacities all patients were treated essentially the same. The following event recounted by an upper staff member reflects the basic concept of equal treatment that line staff employed:

> US–02: When she was wheeled onto the unit, the charge nurse, I guess, saw her coming down. And Sally Walters had her sunglasses on. They are prescription glasses. And [the charge nurse] took them off her and said, "We'll have no Greta Garbos here." That started it real bad. Because of that, in Mrs. Walters's little moments of paranoia she thinks that the staff thinks that she thinks that she's better than everybody else and wants more favorite attention.

These restrictions were sometimes enforced by the use of various degrees of physical force.

> Observation: *Two volunteers begin moving patients to the elevator to take them down to the second floor for the movie. Mrs. Donner tries to get out of her wheelchair.*
> VOLUNTEER 1: Now sit down. (sternly)
> Observation: *Volunteer 1 pulls Mrs. Donner back into her chair from behind by her shoulders.*
> MRS. DONNER: What? (surprised)
> VOLUNTEER 1: You're not going anywhere. We're going to take you on the elevator down to the movie.
> Observation: *Volunteer 1 takes Mrs. Donner onto the elevator.*

The unwritten rule that patients should attend activities whenever the staff could arrange for them to do so sometimes was enforced coercively.

> Observation: *I go back down to the TV lounge. There are some patients from the third floor up here for the music group. (Staff member) walks over to Mrs. Owen, who is attempting to leave music therapy, and locks the brakes on her wheelchair.*
> STAFF: We'll be done soon. You stay here.
> MRS. OWEN: I can't go anywhere. (disgustedly)

These and other small restrictions were quite common:

> UNIDENTIFIED PATIENT: Honey, will you take me to the phone? It's just that [my son] hasn't called and I think his wife is in the hospital and they said that she may have to have an operation. . . .
> Note: *This patient had just arrived at this facility.*
> AIDE: I can't do that. You have to wait for a nurse.
> PATIENT: Thank you. (very passively) (twitching and staring down at the floor)

The aide's rationale for denying the patient's request in this instance is unclear; there are other examples in the data of aides allowing patients to use the staff area phone. However, these other examples involved patients who were capable of walking or rolling themselves down the hallway to the phone. Our general observation is that staff frequently defer decisions to upper staff as a means of saving their time and energy.

Interviews with upper staff provided some evidence that institutional control of patients' daily routines was considered an acceptable institutional norm. The following upper staff member was completing a training internship during the data collection.

> OBSERVER: Are there any particular kinds of techniques that you use to get a person that doesn't particularly want to attend, or is not sure that she wants to attend, to come out and do it?
> STAFF: Uh-huh.
> OBSERVER: What do you say to them? Or what do you do?
> STAFF: To some people we just say, "We're just going down there to sing one time, and you're going to go." (laughing)
> OBSERVER: So you don't give them a choice?
> STAFF: No. Some of these people are kind of tried out already. They . . . either my supervisor or the previous interns have found that these people do enjoy it once they get there. But they refuse the whole time. Like if you ask them, "We're having sing-along. Would you like to come?" They'll always say no. But if you get them down there, then they love it.

Some of the routine methods for controlling patient activities reflected the therapeutic goal of keeping patients active.

> Note: *This conversation took place during an admissions tour.*
> UPPER STAFF: Well, we try to provide some structure. They have to get up and dress and go to meals if they can. We just don't let them sit around.
> DAUGHTER: I think that's great.
> WIFE: Oh, yes.
> DAUGHTER: We just can't seem to get him to do much of anything.

It is interesting to note that the family was very supportive of this approach and that the staff member (who frequently said similar things on admissions tours) seemed confident that they would be. Whether family members understood the pressures that staff would use to "keep them busy" is unclear.

Patients' response to these routines varied widely. Interestingly, some patients shared the view that all patients should be treated equally and follow staff-defined rules.

> MRS. OWEN: I didn't get a donut.
> MRS. BENNETT: I saw you. You had cake. You can't have both.

However, among the cognitively intact patients there was considerable resentment of these restrictions, as can be seen in this patient's view of staff's control over her daily routine.

> MS. KOSAK: They're not used to people like me. She (friend) said, "If you were a little more backward, you might get along better and you could cope with it more. But you're too open with it." But I can't help that.
> OBSERVER: Sometimes the staff is not receptive to your comments?
> MS. KOSAK: Sometimes they tell you that you gotta do something. Maybe you don't feel like you can do it that particular day.
> OBSERVER: They want you to do something when you're not in the mood to do it?
> MS. KOSAK: You may not be up to doing it. That's what I mean. . . .

However, the most common response by impaired individuals to staff-imposed structure was no response. This suggests limited patient comprehension of both the specific restriction and the general situation. In the marginal cases, it is unclear whether the absence of objection is a function of cognitive impairment or acceptance of the staff-patient hierarchy.

We observed a few instances in which impaired individuals continued to voice protest in response to staff restrictions, despite a considerable amount of physical handling and redirection by staff. The most frequent objector was a grossly impaired intermediate patient, Mrs. Zelkan, who objected to practically everything. The staff responded to this patient by getting very frustrated, even angry, as seen both in the style of delivery (eg, verbal threats, directives, and physical redirection) and the content of their statements.

> Observation: *An aide comes down to the staff lounge and starts to roll the food cart down the hallway. In a few moments, the partially loaded*

cart is in the television lounge. She then begins to collect trays from the patients in the lounge.
MRS. ZELKAN: No! No! Leave me that stuff! No! I'm not done yet! No! No!
Observation: *[She] was about half-finished with her meal.*
MRS. ZELKAN: No! No! I'm not done! Please give me my tray. I wish [my son] would come!
Observation: *She is crying and squirming in her seat. The aide continues loading trays and taking off patients' bibs.*
MRS. ZELKAN: No! No!
Observation: *She holds on to her bib, refusing to let the aide take it.*
MRS. ZELKAN: I won't do any of it!
AIDE: Then let go. (sounds disgusted)
MRS. ZELKAN: Why! Why!
Observation: *Mrs. Zelkan lets go of the bib. The aide takes it, as well as her tray.*
AIDE: Be quiet!

Some attempts at objection came in the form of passive resistance.

Observation: *Suddenly the fire alarm goes off.*
PAGING: Attention, everyone. 4A hallway west. Attention. 4A hallway west.
Observation: *This residential floor is being evacuated. (Staff) scurries around assuring the residents that this is just a fire drill. She and the monitor on duty knock on residents' doors, telling them that they must evacuate. Then they close all of the doors. Meanwhile, a man with a stop watch and a clipboard stands in the hallway, watching us all. The only resident to stay in his room is John Taylor. He is noncompliant with the evacuation. The monitor goes into his room.*
MONITOR: Everyone has to leave the floor! If you don't leave, I'll have to come back and take you out in a wheelchair.
MR. TAYLOR: So get a wheelchair. (matter-of-factly)
Observation: *She comes out of the room. (to me) Do you know what he said? He said, "Get a wheelchair." She runs to get it.*

Residential Care

Restrictions similar to those imposed on patients were imposed on residents whom the staff thought were cognitively impaired. These restrictions, however, were more likely to be instituted to avoid potential destructive behavior than to increase institutional efficiency.

> MRS. KELLER (resident monitor): She (Lucille) is not permitted to do her hand laundry in that room. She is to go downstairs and wash.
> OBSERVER: Why?
> MRS. KELLER: Because she created a situation where she flooded the pharmacy and thousands of dollars of drugs were destroyed.

Restrictions were also imposed on behaviors that other residents, touring families, or even staff might have find offensive.

> MONITOR: . . . and Mrs. Camden. She thinks she's Lady Godiva! She was doing it again last night. She came up the hall stark ass naked. I said, "Mary, you can't walk the hall naked!" She said, "Oh, I didn't know that." Right. (disgustedly) I took her back down to her room and two minutes later she was up here with no clothes on again. So I took her back down and I said, "Don't you want to put your nightgown on?" She said, "No, if I get cold I'll just put my coat on." And then she pulled out this sealskin coat. . . .

Despite these examples, residents appear to be given much more freedom than patients. This freedom appears to be both a function of the inclusion criteria (residents must be ambulatory to remain in the residence) and the staff's stated desire to preserve residents' independence. In the following example, however, the observer suspects that the convenience of the staff is an additional motive. The resident in this example manifests gross cognitive impairment.

> Observation: *As I talked with Mrs. Camden, Mrs. Miller headed down the hallway and into the third floor lounge. As usual, she was humming. I assume that she's continuing her search for the "baby with the two different feet." According to staff, this resident spends a better part of her days wandering around the second, third, and fourth floors of [the facility] looking for this imaginary baby. Basically, they don't mind her wandering around. First, they think it's good exercise. Second, she can't get too far. Every time she has tried to leave the building, she has been nabbed at the door. I suspect that an additional reason is that whenever this woman is wandering around the building she is out of their hair. Around dinnertime a scouting expedition is sent out. When they catch up with her, they simply point her in the direction of the dining hall. She is the essence of cooperation.*

Conclusion

In sum, the restrictions placed on patients and residents reflect institutional norms. The norms are situation-specific, but focus primarily on physical maintenance, regulatory and in-house policies regarding reimbursement, and the maintenance of institutional routines. In general, residents are subject to far fewer restrictions of behavior than patients. The purpose of these restrictions is primarily either to promote patient safety or physical well-being, or to increase institutional efficiency.

Support for restrictions on patients' behaviors varied across staff groups. Line staff imposed substantial restrictions, some effected via coercion, redirection, and physical restraint; upper staff, on the other hand, were more supportive of patient independence in both theory and practice. Cognitively impaired patients offered little resistance to behavior control, while mildly impaired and intact patients verbalized objections that were seldom translated into action.

NOTES

1. The relationship between liberty and autonomy is a complex one. See Chapter 1. See also Hayworth 1986.

2. It is interesting that Mill makes a rather broad exception to the liberty that he proposes to give to all; "It is, perhaps, hardly necessary to say that this is only meant to apply to human beings in the maturity of their faculties. We are not speaking of children, or of young persons below the age which the law may fix as that of manhood or womanhood. . . . For the same reason, we may leave out of consideration those backward states of society in which the race itself may be considered as in its nonage. . . . Despotism is a legitimate mode of government in dealing with barbarians" (Mill 1955:14). Mill apparently did not consider those who once had "their faculties" and lost them.

3. It also should be pointed out that not all experts in the field of geriatric care believe that restraints prevent injuries from occurring. Experts also criticize the use of restraints because their use further weakens the muscles that are supposed to protect the body from falls. See particularly Evans and Strumpf 1989.

4. As far as we can determine, there is no legal authority for this restriction.

5. One of the problems in the intermediate care facility is that patients' cognitive abilities, and hence ability to behave autonomously, varied widely. The restrictions, however, were applied indiscriminately. Because of institutional bias toward preserving physical health and assumptions regarding patients' lack of autonomy, freedom was often unjustly limited for minimally impaired patients.

6. Questions regarding inequalities in private resources were clearly seen as outside the staff's influence and treated as an external constraint.

7

Activities and Schedules: The Routine of Daily Life

Autonomy in the long-term care context, as we have tried to indicate, is heavily influenced by the institutional structuring of everyday existence. Thus, we need to know the degree to which patients and residents controlled their own routines in the institutions in which they lived and the sorts of choices they had in their day-to-day lives. A good way of looking at that concerns how patients' and residents' time was scheduled and structured.

Temporal Autonomy

All human activity takes place in time. While the "objective time" of the clock and the calendar are relatively modern inventions (Zerubavel 1979, 1981), all activities occur in sequences and, thus, temporarily is an essential aspect of all interactions.

Superficially, it might seem that this aspect of human existence has nothing to do with autonomy. It is beyond our control. As we say, "Time waits for no one." Yet, within its continuous flow, time can be used in many different ways. To begin with, time may be scheduled or it may be unscheduled. More importantly, it may be scheduled by oneself or by others. Whatever the difficulties that people have in scheduling their own time, they have more autonomy in their lives if they control their own time. Being able to control their time allows them to define who they are by controlling what they do at a particular point in time. A trivial example is our ability to control when we get up in the morning. Our conception of ourselves as early risers or night owls is particularly dependent on our ability to control the time of day we choose to get out of bed.

Yet, even within the categories of self-scheduled time versus other-scheduled time, there are substantial differences in autonomy. First, one may have one's time scheduled by others in conformity with one's wishes, eg, the executive whose secretary schedules meetings at the executive's general directions or keeps a schedule book to organize the executive's responsibilities. On the other hand, the prisoner or army private may have schedules made completely at the whim of superiors. Second, schedules may be more or less required. A schedule to pick up one's five-year-old child after school may seem very compelling and almost totally inflexible if the child has no other transportation home. On the other hand, a scheduled plan to watch a TV show with the rest of the family may be cancelled on a whim.[1]

Thus, it is useful to identify two aspects of temporal autonomy in the long-term care facility. First, there is the organization of schedules and the degree to which it is under the patients' control or reflects their choices. Second, there is the flexibility of the schedule as reflected in the ability of the individual patient to make spontaneous choices.

Schedules of Care

There are obvious similarities between the schedules of institutionalized and noninstitutionalized individuals; both serve to regulate the location in time and frequency of events that occur in a person's life. The most noticeable distinction between the two, however, lies in the degree of control afforded individuals over the timing of the various activities that make up their daily schedules.

In order to understand this, one must understand something about the institutional schedule as well as the staff's perceptions of their responsibilities, which we discussed in Chapters 3 and 5. The line staff had a rigid schedule which they did their best to follow in order to complete all of the necessary tasks in the assigned times. In the morning, these tasks included getting patients up in the morning, toileting, bathing, dressing, and feeding them.

> MS. LAUGHREN (an aide): (to observer) Hey, you need to be here in the early morning. That's when things are really hopping.
> OBSERVER: How so?

> Ms. Laughren: We get seven or eight patients and we have to get each of them washed and dressed.

Patients were generally awakened at 7:30 AM and had to be toileted, washed, dressed, and in place for breakfast by 9 AM. This allowed each patient roughly ten to fifteen minutes of staff assistance. Consequently staff felt incapable of allowing patients any flexibility in such decisions as when they would get up; in the interest of institutional efficiency patients were forced to adhere to a pre-established schedule. Further, within the established schedule the order of events was fixed; all patients were awakened, toileted, washed, and finally dressed in sequence.

The lunch and bedtime schedules were also characterized by a lack of flexibility. Lunchtime was scheduled every day from noon to one, varying only on Friday when it was preceded by a 15-minute "happy hour." The morning activities were performed in reverse order in the evening; patients had dinner at five, followed by the assistance of aides in undressing, washing, toileting, and going to bed.

The overall time frame and sequence of events was seldom negotiable. There was no variation in the location, timing, or duration of meals. Patients scheduled to eat in the dining hall who chose to stay on the units, for example, missed their meals. One patient, in particular, enjoyed a 1 PM soap opera. In order to avoid missing the show (as a result of not being allowed to come back up from the dining hall early), this patient regularly skipped lunch.

Patients eating on the units were allowed one hour to eat; regardless of whether they were finished, their trays were removed at the end of the hour. Likewise, patients transported to the dining hall were not permitted to leave that area until the dining period was over.

> Observation: *The dining period was approximately 45 minutes long. Some residents wandered in rather casually and seated themselves. The patients were mostly rolled in. With the exception of Ms. Viancia, however, everyone stayed seated until it was announced that the dining period was over. Then they trailed to the elevator and went (or were taken) to their respective floors.*

Beyond one attempt by Ms. Viancia to leave the dining hall early, there were no other attempts at deviation noted. It is notable, though, that the attempted deviation from routine by Ms. Viancia was met with immediate, effective staff resistance in view of all the patients, as described in Chapter 6.

The times for rising and going to bed were no more flexible.

Note: *Post dinner, 6:30* PM
Observation: *She (patient) let me know that she was tired and wished she could go to bed . . . but that she usually wasn't allowed to go to bed until about 7:30.*

In spite of the rigidity of the patients' schedules, review of the scheduled activities cited above suggests that patients have control of the majority of their time. A closer examination of the ways in which patients spend the "unscheduled" portion of their days, however, suggests otherwise.

Most intermediate and skilled care patients, particularly those restrained in wheelchairs or geri-chairs, spent the better part of their days parked in front of any of a variety of facility television sets. These sets were almost always playing at a volume that made conversation extremely difficult. There was little verbal indication of patients' feelings about this activity, although there was little indication of enthusiasm.

Note: *Breakfast.*
Observation: *There are six patients sitting in the third-floor television lounge. All appear to be asleep. Breakfast trays are scattered around. The television is running a talk show.*
Note: *11:22* A.M.
Observation: *I get off the elevator on the third floor. There are several women in wheelchairs sitting by a low table in front of the television set.*
Note: *2:45* PM
Observation: *As I get off the elevator on the fourth floor I almost run into a woman sitting in a wheelchair. She doesn't appear to notice me. Her eyes are glued to the television set. There are three other patients in wheelchairs sitting in front of the table by the TV. There are several others sitting around in chairs looking [dazed]. The volume on the television is a little lower than normal.*
Note: *5:34* PM
Observation: . . . *[on] the fourth floor . . . the TV is still running. There are a few people sitting in front of the TV. All of them are in wheelchairs or geri-chairs. They don't appear to be watching the television or interacting with each other. They look veged out. . . . There are six patients sitting in the television lounge. One has a walker; the other five are in wheelchairs. Three of the wheelchair patients are women. The television is running, but no one is looking at it.*
TV: "Our next puzzle is a thing." (game show)

As seen above, the lounge televisions generally ran throughout the day and early evening; this was as true on weekends and holidays as it was on weekdays. About the only times that the lounge televisions were turned off was during activities in the lounges. Then, as seen below, they were immediately turned back on.

> Note: *Music therapy in the fourth floor lounge has just ended.*
> Observation: *The music therapist puts her guitar and music paraphernalia away. She turns on the TV and pushes tables and chairs back into place.*
> TV: ". . . that's one way he can make his heart healthier: by lowering the cholesterol."

Further, while a few patients, primarily those who did not have televisions in their rooms, occasionally came to the lounges to watch television, for the most part the patients in these lounges were cognitively impaired and immobile. The sporadic and limited nature of the patients' cognitive abilities limited inter-patient conversations. Attempts at spontaneous conversation were made even more difficult by the television's volume.

> Note: *Fourth-floor television lounge following dinner.*
> MRS. ZELKAN: (whining) I wanted to get another look at my tray. (her dinner tray was taken before she was finished)
> MRS. BENNETT: I don't have it.
> MRS. ZELKAN: No. I don't know what they have. They took things I didn't have.
> MRS. BENNETT: I finished eating pretty good.
> MRS. ZELKAN: Nurse, honey. Please come here a minute!
> MRS. KRAMER: Honey! (singing)
> Note: *An aide is passing through the lounge. She does not respond.*
> Observation: *Mrs. Mitnick grabs at Kerry Kennedy (aide). She does not get hold of her.*
> MRS. OWEN: You never did be good, did you?
> MRS. BENNETT: No. (shaking head)
> MRS. KRAMER: Oh, oh, oh, oh, oh, oh, oh. . . . (singing with powdered sugar all over her mouth)
> TV: I'm Hank B." (news)
> MRS. ZELKAN: Nurse, please come here honey!
> MRS. MITNICK: Ugh, ugh, ugh. . . .
> Observation: *Mrs. Mitnick begins beating rhythmically on the wheelchair table. She is using her fist.*
> MRS. ZELKAN: You want a drop of tea or give it to me?

MRS. BENNETT: No.
MRS. MITNICK: Ugh, ugh, ugh. . . .
Observation: *She begins shaking her geri-chair desk.*
MRS. OWEN: Don't do that.
MRS. KRAMER: Well, I have to.
MRS. OWEN: Why?
MRS. MITNICK: Ugh, ugh, ugh. . . .
MRS. ZELKAN: I'd just like to tell Bob (son) about that!
Observation: *Mrs. Mitnick is now grunting, with her eyes closed. She is also rocking back and forth in her wheelchair.*

Although it was certainly practical to group these patients in one large area since it allowed staff to check on them easily from a distance, it further restricted their already limited ability to initiate activity. First, these patients were, for the most part, surrounded by other impaired patients with whom they could not have meaningful interactions. Second, they were seldom able to get the attention of staff members unless staff chose to come into the area. While this allowed staff freedom from the repetitive requests of impaired patients, it limited patients' access to staff who could move them or attempt to engage them in meaningful interactions. Third, the din of the constantly running televisions made conversation of any kind difficult. Finally, by relegating these physically impaired patients to this communal area without any consideration of their wishes, patients were denied access to personal possessions and the privacy of their own rooms.

This pervasive form of patient management resulted in impaired patients spending their days immobile in front of a television with limited opportunities for personal growth or social activities. In this context, it is clear that most patients had very little say over where or how they spent most of their waking hours. Although few patients complained about being left unattended in these lounges for long periods of time, some did.

Note: *Fourth-floor lounge.*
MRS. WILSON: (to observer, in one of her few lucid moments) Please ask them (staff) where Mrs. Wilson (the patient) was all day. I'd just like to know. I'd just be very interested in knowing where they thought I was all day. (sarcastically)

Those patients who were bedfast were limited to interacting with various line staff during the performance of their care duties, interacting with guests, and participating in an occasional one-on-one session with the music or recreational therapist. The remainder of their days were spent listening to television in their rooms or lying in silence. However, the ability of these patients to initiate activity appeared to be minimal and, consequently, there is little reason to believe that these patients would have been able to structure their time even if permitted to do so.

At the other extreme, cognitively intact, mobile patients were constrained only by the scheduling of meals and in-house recreational events. Most of these patients (although there were few on either unit) voiced no objections to the scheduling of meals, and reported being relatively satisfied with the nature and scheduling of recreational events. Several, including one wheelchair-bound cerebral palsy patient, regularly scheduled their own off-grounds recreation.

Scheduled Breaks in the Routine—Weekly Activities

Patients' days were not spent exclusively in their rooms or in front of TV sets. Common events, such as recreational activities, were scheduled at least weekly. Indeed, a calendar of events was posted on the bulletin board weekly, letting everyone who could read see what activities were being offered. One week's calendar looked like this:

Sunday
10 AM Communion on the units
1 PM Church in the Common Lounge

Monday
11 AM "Good Old Days" (trip down memory lane)
2 PM Flower arranging

Tuesday
11 AM Sing along (music therapy)
1 PM recreation groups (games . . .)
2 PM (choice) crafts or outside trip

Wednesday
11 AM group walk outside
2 PM bowling

Thursday
10 AM Mass
2 PM crafts

Friday
10:30 AM exercise group
11:00 AM "Musical Memories"
2:30 PM Bingo

Saturday
11 AM Current Events (discussion group)

These activities were popular with families, who were commonly shown these boards during the course of admissions tours.

> Observation: *US–05 stops by the activity board. She explains it, and points out a number of the activities going on this week. Both family members seem impressed.*
> US–05: This is the activity schedule.
> Observation: *She stops in front of it. The two women scan it.*
> FIRST WOMAN: That's nice.
> US–05: You see they have booze and gambling on Friday. . . . (referring to Happy Hour and bingo)
> SECOND WOMAN: (laughing) They're really bad here. That's nice. (laughs)

Most patients indicated that they enjoyed these recreational activities and gave no indication of discontent with any aspects of their scheduling. The patient in the example below complained vociferously about almost all aspects of the institution, but she attended (and enjoyed) almost all available recreational activities.

> OBSERVER: What kind of things do you like here . . . at [facility]?
> MS. KOZAK: The music.
> OBSERVER: Do you like to sing or do you like to listen?
> MS. KOZAK: Both. (pause) And I like creative cooking.
> OBSERVER: So you like to cook and you go to music therapy. And what else do you like to do?
> MS. KOZAK: Movies and shopping.

It is important to note that most of the activities offered were available only to a limited number of patients. Many of the patients were too physically or mentally impaired to participate in the recreational activities. Thus, many of the bedridden patients were not able to enjoy scheduled recreational activities. Moreover, some activities, especially those that involved leaving the institution, required a large staff-to-patient ratio and were thus limited to a few patients at a time. The times, locations, and duration of these activities were structured to fit into the staff schedule which, in turn, was partially determined by the number of facilities and patients that upper staff were expected to serve.

> MUSIC THERAPIST: OK. Tuesday morning is the social group at [facility 2] for the Med/Surg patients. Then Tuesday afternoons we spend seeing one-on-ones at [facility 2]. Wednesday mornings is choir for the gerontology here. Then, let's see . . . Wednesdays. Oh, we went to see one-on-ones at [facility 2] again. And then we came back to hospice to see the people that I hadn't seen on Monday. On Thursday mornings I'm here and then back to [facility 2]. Friday mornings I do a small group. There are small groups done on three floors.

Thus, both upper staff and patients were "locked" into pre-determined schedules that dictated which recreational activities would be offered when and to whom.

Although most patients seemed to enjoy scheduled activities, the decision to participate in weekly recreational events was not always voluntary. Many patients were "strongly encouraged" to attend activities.

> US–14: Are you coming to the hymn sing?
> MS. BENNETT: Please don't. (crying and probably in one of her periodic demented phases)
> US–14: OK.
> MS. BENNETT: Please don't. Please don't. I just can't take it anymore.
> US–14: How about I take you down? You'll enjoy yourself.

The upper staff sought to maximize participation by patients in activities based on the notion that keeping patients active was in their best interest and that, left to structure their own time, patients would not put it to good use. Thus, staff frequently attempted to persuade patients that participation was "for their own good." This is a classical example of a conflict between beneficence and autonomy values made more interesting by the fact that the staff were trying to promote some of the very capabilities that permit autonomous activity (Collopy 1986).

Since patients attending activities were the responsibility of upper staff for the duration of the activity, line staff tended to see such activities as a chance to get patients off the unit and, thus, get a break from their workload. Consequently, the line staff were also strongly inclined to "encourage" patients to go to scheduled activities whether they wanted to or not. As seen in earlier sections, unsuccessful attempts at persuasion by line staff were occasionally followed by physical redirection and coercion.

Participation in specially scheduled activities like holiday parties and other ritual events appeared, however, to be genuinely at the discretion of the participants, regardless of their residence or competence. For example, attendance by patients at the Valentine party cited below was completely voluntary, even for patients who were substantially cognitively compromised. Some patients who attended this party rarely left their units, while other, more active patients declined to attend.

> Note: *Valentine party.*
> Observation: *I take the steps down to the second floor to see what's going on at the Valentine party. [The recreational therapist] is on the microphone, reading Valentine poems written by various patients. The room is full of patients, including many of those who normally eat on the units. The patients are seated around tables covered with red tablecloths. On each table is a bouquet of red and white carnations and containers of Valentine candy. . . . After the poetry reading, [the music therapist] takes over and plays the piano as she leads the group in a rendition of "Let Me Call You Sweetheart." . . . Most of the patients appear to be at least trying to sing. Volunteers circulate among them, encouraging them to participate.*

In general, then, a variety of collective recreational activities were offered to patients at varying intervals. Overall, the times of infrequent activities were dictated by the calendar, while the locations, times, and durations of the more frequent activities were dictated by the availability of facility areas and staff. Depending on their cognitive abilities, patients had almost complete control over their participation in the relatively infrequent events (eg, parties), and somewhat less control over their participation in the more frequent activities (eg, hymn sings, bingo). For the most part, families indicated their approval of both the general concept of keeping people active and the range of activities offered. Most patients indicated that they enjoyed these activities although it is unclear how important their wishes were to staff's scheduling of these events.

Residence Routines and Schedules

The residents' schedule was largely self-directed. In general, residents had the same calendar of activities available to them that the patients did, and they constituted a substantial portion of the attendees at most functions. In some cases, residents were encouraged by staff to participate in these functions.

> OBSERVER: What does Kathryn (resident) spend the better part of her time doing?
> MS. OLSON: (resident monitor): Walking and asking questions. Asking you when she's going home, and eating out of our kitchen. . . . That's it. I have said, "They are playing bingo downstairs." She'll say that she doesn't like bingo. I'll tell her to just go and be with other people. "You know, I wouldn't go and play bingo (just to play bingo) either. But why don't you go down?" And she'll just say, "No, I don't think so." She goes occasionally. And she may go to the movies. Or walk.

The residents expressed varying degrees of interest in the scheduled activities. Kathryn (the subject of the resident monitor's comment) told one of our interviewers:

> OBSERVER: What will you do with yourself until then? Until you can go home?
> KATHRYN: Read a lot. Here is a Reader's Digest. I read this. This is a boring place.

On the other hand, Mrs. Segal (another resident) viewed matters very differently.

> OBSERVER: How do you like it so far?
> MRS. SEGAL: I like it very well. They have activities for you and I can still go out. . . .
> OBSERVER: Which ones do you enjoy the most?
> MRS. SEGAL: . . . we have bowling and, of course, every Wednesday we are supposed to go. . . . Now tonight they have what is called table games. They play Family Feud or trivia or something. And then Tuesday night an AARP group, I think, from West Hills. . . . Once a month they come and we play bingo at night. I always go to that.

Beyond the encouragement from the resident monitors to get involved in activities, the residents largely determined their own schedules. While residents were required to go to the dining hall at regularly scheduled times to get their meals rather than having them brought to the residence, they were free to eat their meals outside the institution.

Resident monitors often helped residents with various ADLs. For example, some of the residents could not bathe themselves without help. However, help with ADLs was not done on a fixed schedule, but at the mutual convenience of the resident and the monitor.

> MRS. MILLER (a registered nurse): They are independent as far as doing their showers. They can do that themselves.
> OBSERVER: You don't have to help with bathing at all?
> MRS. MILLER: There are some you do and some that you don't. Ms. Brown takes her own shower every morning. Occasionally, she will ask you to wash her back and then that is the extent of it for her. Some of the people require assistance in bathing. . . . Some people need assistance with medications.

Conclusion

In summary, the scheduling of routine activities and the amount of structure that was imposed was strongly related to the cognitive and physical abilities of the individuals. At one extreme were the moderately to severely demented patients who spent their days in the lounge with the TV blaring and whose daily routines, such as eating and sleeping, were highly structured by the staff. At the other extreme were the residents who, cognitively capable or not, were largely allowed to spend their time as they liked.

NOTES

1. Another factor that has important implications for autonomy is the meaning of the scheduled time to the patient. All other things being equal, the more central the block of time (or the activity being conducted during that time) is to an individual the more important it is to a person's autonomy whether the time is self- or other-scheduled (Hayworth 1986).

8

Interaction Patterns and Autonomy

Humans beings spend large amounts of their time interacting with each other. Many of the things we value involve interaction patterns and/or are available to us only through interaction with other human beings. This is particularly true if one is old and physically disabled in some way.

If we view autonomy as consistency and thus as critically intertwined with one's current commitments and future projects, patterns of interaction are important aspects of autonomy. Such theorists as Katz (1984) and Burt (1979) have even argued that the central goal of the autonomy doctrine of informed consent is the modification of the patterns of interaction between doctors and patients.

What does interaction in these settings look like? Do we see the sort of autonomy-enhancing interactions that Katz sought, in which the patient and caregiver work together to develop the patient's understanding of the issues in care provision and the caregiver's understanding of the things in the patient's life that he or she values? Or, on the contrary, do we see interactions that demean one or both parties in the setting and prevent the clarification, expression, and implementation of patient choices? Do the interactions provide support for the patient to function as an independent agent or serve to make the patient even more dependent on staff?

A related issue is the nature of the interaction among the patients. It is easy to imagine that patients could provide a significant support group for each other's autonomous relationship with the staff and the outside world. Indeed, there is considerable literature that seeks to demonstrate that supportive interactions among patients can provide a significant aid in dealing with the difficult features of decision-making in medical care

(Gartner and Reissman 1977, Lieberman 1979, Gottlieb 1982). On the other hand, as we noted in Chapter 5, the normative patterns surrounding the sick role lead friends and relatives of patients to encourage passivity and compliance in a variety of situations. Lidz et al. (1984) have even reported that some patients encourage their associates to comply with the very treatments that they themselves refused. Thus, the patterns of interaction among patients and residents should be of considerable interest.

Staff-Patient Interaction Patterns

Day-to-day interaction between staff and patients consisted primarily of requests by patients for assistance, information, or permission from various staff members and the responses from staff. We coded these three different types of requests separately, and they do differ somewhat.[1] Requests for information generally required only that the staff give a verbal response, while giving permission for, or agreeing to assist with, an activity generally necessitated a greater effort on the part of staff. For example, giving a patient permission to go to bed early required staff to assist the patient in preparing for bed. However, since requests for information were generally made in conjunction with requests for assistance or permission, all these requests can be analyzed together.

In general, most requests by patients related to help with ADLs, and addressed such things as requests for water, to be moved, and to be taken to the bathroom. Some of these seemed to exemplify a cooperative and mutually exploratory mode of interaction.

> Note: *The patient in the following example is physically impaired, including her speech, but mentally intact.*
> Ms. Graves: Uh . . . uh. . . .
> Observation: *Ms. Graves is parked close in front of the television set. Ms. Laughren (an aide) walks over to see what she wants.*
> Ms. Laughren: What?
> Observation: *Ms. Laughren sits down in front of Ms. Graves, where the patient can see her. She gives the patient her total attention.*
> Ms. Graves: (says something that I can't make out)
> Ms. Laughren: You want more water?
> Ms. Graves: (says something else that I can't make out)
> Ms. Laughren: You still have half a glass.
> Ms. Graves: (says something else that I can't understand)
> Ms. Laughren: (laughing) I'll get you two more if that's what you want.

While some requests were honored and others were not, the amount of cognitive impairment of the patient seemed to be a dominant factor in determining which requests would be honored. Most requests by cognitively intact patients were honored although sometimes it was necessary for patients to be persistent. In the few examples where staff denied requests, intact patients attempted to act alone.

> US–15: Ms. Kosak is contented now. The other day . . . we had a farewell for (administrator) before she left, . . . It really was just for staff. Ms. Kosak went to her cupboard and said that she needed someone to help her change her clothes so she could go down to the party. This is like our lunch hour, and a really bad time. So I said, "I'm sorry, Ms. Kosak, You just can't take our time right now to do that now." So here Ms. Kosak went in and changed herself (and went to the party)

In cases like this, in which requests by cognitively intact patients were denied, the denials appeared to reflect the unavailability of staff or conflicting schedules. Here again, as we saw in the last chapter, routine scheduled activities such as feeding or bathing generally took precedence over specific individual requests. When staff felt that they did not have time, it generally meant that the routine care schedule required them to perform another task at that point in time.

The large majority of requests in our notes, however, came from cognitively impaired patients (79%), and nearly half of them came from one patient, Ms. Zelkan. Some were directed toward specific staff or family members, while others were repeatedly asked of whomever was passing by. Most of these requests, particularly those made by Ms. Zelkan, were simply ignored. The following excerpt from the field notes describes interactions in the patient lounge and shows how Ms. Zelkan's requests were dealt with and suggests why.

> Observation: *Ms. Biggs (nurse) comes out of the medication room with the cart. She stops by the time cards.*
> Ms. ZELKAN: (yelling from the television lounge) Nurse! Nurse! Are you cold? Are you cold? (pause) I am, too. . . . Are you all right, honey? Have you got what you need?
> Observation: *Ms. Blitz (patient) continues to snore. Ms. Martine (patient), parked all the way down the hallway, continues to stare in silence.*
> Ms. ZELKAN: Mom, please come here!

Observation: *Mr. Anderson (patient) and his wife walk down the hallway.*
Ms. ZELKAN: Are you working, honey? Honey!
Observation: *An aide takes Ms. Gartner (patient) from her place in the hallway into her room.*

Ms. Zelkan's cognitive state and that of other impaired patients played a large part in their requests being denied or ignored; most of the requests for information alone from this group, for example, indicated a lack of orientation to time or place.

Ms. VIANCIA (patient): It's Sunday, isn't it?
Ms. HARTMAN: (an aide): No, Ms. Viancia. It's Tuesday.
Ms. VIANCIA: Is it?
Ms. HARTMAN: Yes.

As with the cognitively intact patients, many of the requests by impaired patients focused on requests for a deviation from the standard institutional routine and were thus typically denied.

Ms. ZELKAN: Nurse! Come here! Where's my coffee?
Ms. BAKER (an aide): (yells from down the hallway) You'll get it when you get your dinner!
Note: *Ms. Viancia is sitting in the hallway outside of her room. It is mid-evening. This patient was invariably the last to be put to bed on this unit because of her difficulty in sleeping through the night. She often requested to be put to bed shortly after dinner.*
Observation: *Ms. Hartman (an aide) comes out of room 3013 and goes down to the linen room by Ms. Viancia.*
Ms. VIANCIA: (to Ms. Hartman) Could I sleep in that room? (pointing to her room)
Observation: *There is no response from Ms. Hartman.*
Ms. VIANCIA: Would you put me in there?
Observation: *There is no response from Ms. Hartman. Ms. Hartman comes back out of the linen room, goes down the hallway, and into a different patient room.*

When the requests of cognitively impaired patients were responded to, they were generally denied.

Ms. ZELKAN: (to aide) Take me out of here. (referring to the gerichair in which she is restrained)

Ms. KENNEDY: I can't do that.
Ms. ZELKAN: Why?
Ms. KENNEDY: You have to stay in the chair.
Ms. ZELKAN: No. (crying)

Other requests were responded to affirmatively by staff, but with the condition that they would be honored when possible within the normal routine. This generally necessitated postponement, often until the next day or week.

Note: *This is the end of a music therapy session.*
Observation: *Nurse Biggs begins rounds with the medication cart. The music therapists circulate around the remaining patients, shaking hands and asking them how they like the music. "You Made Me Love You" comes on the stereo. Ms. Woodland asks one music therapist if they could hear another record.*
MUSIC THERAPIST: No, not now. But next time.
Observation: *She takes off the record.*

Still others, while not flatly denied, were postponed until an unspecified time when the required staff effort would not compromise the regular routine.

Observation: . . . *meanwhile an aide walks down the hallway. Ms. Viancia spots her.*
Ms. VIANCIA: Will you take me to the bathroom?
Ms. HARTMAN: Not right now, Ms. Viancia.
Ms. VIANCIA: Then when?
Observation: *The aide continues down the hallway. There is no response.*

Some requests from impaired patients were granted immediately. This was most likely when the staff thought that the request was reasonable, they had not granted this same request for this patient recently, they were not busy with other patients, or the request took no time to fulfill. For example, the approval of Mr. Friedman's request for use of the telephone did not necessitate assistance by staff.

Observation: *Mr. Friedman rolls down the hallway and asks an aide for the use of the (staff) phone. He takes it, dials, and talks to someone.*

Other requests were granted with the understanding that no further assistance would be granted on this matter in the near future.

> Ms. ZELKAN: Give me a towel! (for use as a bib)
> STAFF: Will you keep it on?
> Ms. ZELKAN: If you say so.

Requests from patients were most likely to be honored when they could be met in the time allotted for that particular patient, and did not require staff to deviate from their normal routine.

> Observation: *Ms. Brosky (an aide) walks up to Ms. Zelkin who is still sitting in the hallway.*
> Ms. BROSKY: Hello, Ms. Zelkan.
> Observation: *Ms. Brosky ties a bib on Ms. Zelkan.*
> Ms. ZELKAN: Will you please leave the door partly closed?
> Observation: *Ms. Brosky goes over to the patient's door, and pulls it part-way shut.*

As can be seen, staff did not respond to many of the requests of the cognitively impaired patients, and when they did it was often to deny or delay them. The most successful technique that impaired patients used when their requests had been ignored or denied was simple persistence. When patients were persistent and requests only minimally inconvenient, staff were inclined to acquiesce rather than put up with the hassle of repeated requests.

> Note: *Ms. Viancia was restrained in a geri-chair with a desk attached to the front, and did not "need" to be moved up to the table to eat.*
> Observation: *They seem to be waiting for dinner.*
> Ms. HARTMAN: (an aide) walks into the lounge. Ms. Viancia spots her.
> Ms. VIANCIA: Put me here, please!
> Observation: *Ms. Viancia gestures to the place at the large table where she would like to sit. Ms. Hartman does not pay attention, going on to another patient.*
> Ms. VIANCIA: Turn me around!
> Observation: *No response from Ms. Hartman.*
> Ms. VIANCIA: Please, turn me around!
> Ms. HARTMAN: Wait a minute, Ms. Viancia.
> Observation: *Ms. Hartman continues to move other patients close to the table in preparation for dinner.*

Ms. Viancia: Will you turn me around? (emphatically)
Observation: *Another aide (Ms. Marshall) walks into the lounge. She says "Wait a minute, Ms. Viancia." This aide moves several other patients near the table.*
Ms. Viancia: Turn me around, please! (growing increasingly upset)
Observation: *Ms. Hartman moves her up to the table.*
Ms. Viancia: This will be okay.
Observation: *Ms. Hartman leaves the lounge, looking at me and rolling her eyes.*

Interestingly, although patients had very little leverage to get staff to comply with their requests, the same was true of staff. Although, of course, staff could control the mobility of those patients restrained in geri- or wheelchairs and many other features of patient activities simply by their greater physical abilities, cooperation from patients was not easily obtained. Patients often did not cooperate or participate in the activities in which staff wanted them to participate.

Note: *Ms. Woodland (a patient) was restrained in a geri-chair and left in the room where the music therapy group was meeting. She was not participating in the group.*
Observer: Why aren't you in the music group? (referring to the five patients participating)
Ms. Woodland: Because I don't want to be.
Observer: You don't like music?
Ms. Woodland: Oh, I like music. Just not the way they play it.

As we have seen in other contexts, the upper staff responded to patients' requests differently than did line staff. Although there are relatively few examples of requests to upper staff that we observed directly, those examples we have show that upper staff handled requests in a less confrontational and more supportive manner than line staff.

Note: *The cognitive status of the patient in the following example is unknown.*
Observation: *A physical therapist helps the man back to his wheelchair. Meanwhile, another physical therapist continues to stand in front of the patient sitting beside me.*
PT–1: OK, Mr. Owen (patient). Lift your legs.
Mr. Owen: Where are we going?
PT–1: Is another walk okay?

> MR. OWEN: Can't I rest a bit?
> PT–1: OK, we'll walk after you rest.

Upper staff appeared to handle cognitively impaired patients in much the same way; patients were accorded much more say in the relationship even when their requests were not acceded to.

> Note: *Ms. Viancia was a grossly impaired patient who believed that she was still teaching a foreign language in a local high school.*
> Observation: *US–19 comes back down the hallway from the staff area. . . . Ms. Viancia addresses [her].*
> MS. VIANCIA: Can you take me home tonight?
> US–19: I'm not sure that I can answer that. Can we talk about it tomorrow at breakfast?
> MS. VIANCIA: Do you mean I'm going to have to miss a day of school?
> US–19: Are you worried about that?
> MS. VIANCIA: They just don't care about me.
> US–19: They don't care about you being here?
> MS. VIANCIA: I'm just sick about it and I don't know what I can do.
> US–19: I can understand that. Can we talk about it tomorrow?
> MS. VIANCIA: Can you take me to my room?
> US–19: Yes.
> MS. VIANCIA: Where is it?
> US–19: Well . . . how about if I help you find it?
> Observation: *US–19 pushes Ms. Viancia away from the table and rolls her down the hallway.*

It is important to note, however, that upper staff was in a better position to provide individualized attention to patients. In fact, not bound by the same rigid routine as line staff, upper staff were often free to provide this attention at their own convenience, and in return received considerable positive feedback from both line staff and patients.

Probably the most important point about these interactions is not the dramatic one, that patient requests are so often ignored, but the mundane one, that the interaction overwhelmingly consists of unidirectional requests. Status, independence and power come from being able to grant requests of others. Subjugation and dependence come from needing to ask for help. These are elemental truths of any system of political power and it applies here. The system of care is so structured, at this institution and every other public care facility that we are aware of, that those cared for have nothing to give to the caregivers except their subservience.

Staff-Resident Interactions

Interaction between staff and residents differed from that of staff and patients in that residents rarely asked staff to grant requests of any kind.[2] Rather, the resident monitors and nurses routinely asked if residents would like help with activities (eg, bathing, dressing, etc.). These interactions seem to reflect the difference between both patient and resident roles and the temporal structure of skilled and intermediate and residential units. The few examples in our data of requests by residents for assistance involved only cognitively impaired residents. There are no examples of requests being ignored; rather, resident monitors and nurses appeared to go to great lengths to understand exactly what these residents wanted and to comply with their requests.

> Observation: *Mrs. Miller (a resident) comes out of the television room. She's waving an orange above her head.*
> MRS. MILLER: Yoo hoo! Yoo hoo!
> Observation: *Ms. Lee (a registered nurse) walks down to see what she wants.*
> MRS. MILLER: Can you give this . . . well, you know . . . to Marie? You know she has those young ones at home.
> MS. LEE: I'm not sure who you're talking about.
> MRS. MILLER: You know. It's the one that I usually bring things up for. You know. The one with all the little ones at home.
> MS. LEE: Do you mean Ms. Sedge?
> MRS. MILLER: Yes. You know, the one with the little ones at home. I want her to take this with her.
> MS. LEE: Ms. Sedge doesn't have any kids.
> MRS. MILLER: Yes. Yes. I want her to have this.
> Observation: *Mrs. Miller is gesturing toward the cart in the hallway piled high with cleaning supplies.*
> MS. LEE: Do you mean Darlene? The cleaning woman. Whoops! The person from environmental services?
> MRS. MILLER: Huh?
> MS. LEE: (yelling) Do you mean Darlene? (gesturing to the cleaning cart).
> MRS. MILLER: Yes! This is for her little ones at home.
> MS. LEE: (taking the orange) That's very nice of you. I'll give it to her.
> MRS. MILLER: Yes. Yes.

The monitors' attempts to honor the requests of cognitively impaired residents is paralleled in their interactions with intact residents. In the following example, despite the staff's wish that this resident (as well as others) would take her medications on a regular basis, the monitors respected Mrs. Pletz's desire to decide for herself when she required medication.

> Note: *Interview with resident monitor.*
> RM: Mrs. Pletz can regulate her own medication the way she wants. When she decides she doesn't want to take something, she just doesn't take it. If you give it to her she just throws it out.

Patient/Patient Interactions

If staff-patient interactions consisted primarily of requests and responses or nonresponses, what did patient/patient interactions look like? After all, other patients were the main group of human beings surrounding any particular patient. It might seem that, while the staff's view of patients and their needs and desires were deeply embedded in the medical model, patients might be more inclined to know each other as complex human beings and thus support a more diverse set of wants and activities on the part of their colleagues. Indeed, in our initial proposal for this research we suggested that interaction among patients might prove a major mechanism to support autonomy. It was with this in mind that we analyzed the patient/patient interactions.

On the surface, most of these interactions[3] seem irrelevant to our theoretical interests. Rather than providing evidence of patients either supporting or discouraging attempts at autonomous behavior by other patients, the majority of these interactions consist simply of casual conversation about such innocuous subjects as the weather or the dinner menu.

> Note: *Ms. Bennett and Ms. Florence have just finished dinner in the television lounge.*
> Ms. Bennett: Wasn't that just awful?
> Ms. Florence: I couldn't eat that pepper.
> Ms. Bennett: I didn't like that coffee, either.
> Ms. Florence: They just can't make it right.
> Ms. Bennett: Yeah.

Not all interactions were of such an impersonal nature. Below, two patients discuss the state of their health.

> Ms. Edwards: And how are you getting along dear?
> Mrs. Ruth: OK.

Ms. Edwards: Really, dear?
Mrs. Ruth: I'm OK. How are things for you?
Ms. Edwards: Well, things are going pretty good.

The interactions above took place between intact and mildly impaired individuals. At the other extreme, severely impaired patients, while following turn-taking rules, seemed barely to be responding to each other.

Ms. Zelkan: Will you have a little lunch?
Ms. Kramer: . . . Yes. (singing her response)
Ms. Zelkan: When?
Ms. Kramer: Yes. (singing)
Ms. Zelkan: (starting to cry) But I don't have it ready.
Ms. Kramer: That's okay, honey.
Ms. Zelkan: When do you want it?
Ms. Kramer: OK, honey. (singing it)
Ms. Zelkan: Are you okay, honey?
Ms. Kramer: Yes, honey. (singing it)
Ms. Zelkan: (to observer) Will you be with me until I get it ready?
Ms. Kramer: Yes. (singing it)
Mr. McLaughlin: Aaaaaahhhhh. . . .

Most interactions between moderately impaired patients were only a little clearer in focus, often highlighting their lack of orientation and containing little, if anything, that might provide support for autonomous behavior.

Ms. Viancia: What day is it?
Ms. Kazmeric: I think it's Saturday.
Ms. Viancia: Is it Sunday or Monday?
Ms. Kazmeric: Maybe Monday.
Observation: *There is a brief pause.*
Mrs. Silverman: Isn't tomorrow Christmas?
Observer: Yes, it is.
Observation: *Several patients appear to ponder this question.*
Ms. Viancia: I don't know.

The majority of patient/patient interactions are quite similar to the ones shown above. A few interactions between demented patients appear on the surface to be supportive of autonomy.

Note: *These are two permanently placed individuals living in the intermediate section of the mixed unit.*
Ms. Viancia: I have a key to my house, but now I don't know where it is.
Ms. Kazmeric: Maybe if you look for it you can find it.
Ms. Viancia: I don't know what to do.
Ms. Kazmeric: You know, it will just fall out of your pocket or something.
Ms. Viancia: I don't have the key to get into my house because I figured he'd (patient's deceased uncle) always be there.
Ms. Kazmeric: Well, if I were you I'd just go over there with some friends and I'd just ring the bell and then I'd just see what happens.
Ms. Viancia: Oh, I'm so upset I just don't know what to do. (agitated)
Ms. Kazmeric: Well, that's understandable . . . but you couldn't have done anything.
Ms. Viancia: Will you go up there with me?
Ms. Kazmeric: Okay.
Ms. Viancia: I thought I had the keys to my house with me and now I know I don't.
Ms. Kazmeric: Well, don't worry about it.
Ms. Viancia: But I do. . . . The lawyer's right down at the corner.
Ms. Kazmeric: Is he?
Ms. Viancia: Yes.
Ms. Kazmeric: Then why don't you ask him if he has the key?
Ms. Viancia: I would, unless it's going to take a whole day. What day is it?

There is, then, some evidence of patients appearing to support autonomous behavior by other patients. However, for all practical purposes this support is not relevant to reality-based activity. Ms. Viancia's actual situation was totally different than she portrayed it and Ms. Kazmeric was unlikely to leave the facility for any purpose.

In theory, interaction with cognitively intact patients might help impaired patients with reality-based behaviors. However, there were few examples of intact patients interacting with impaired patients and most were brief, and were terminated by the intact patients at the first sign of confusion.

Note: *A meal has just been finished. Ms. Florence stops beside Ms. Zelkan on her way down the hall to her room.*
Ms. Florence: It looks like you did a good job eating.

Ms. ZELKAN: No, they didn't come out on time.
Ms. FLORENCE: Uh-huh.
Observation: *Ms. Florence continues down the hall.*

In general, intact patients appeared to find interacting with cognitively compromised patients frustrating. Even the mildly impaired patients disliked being in the presence of those most severely impaired.

Note: *These patients are impaired: Ms. Zelkan severely, Ms. Donner moderately, and Ms. Bennett mildly. They are sitting in the television lounge.*
Ms. ZELKAN: I'm sorry, Dad, for everything I did!
Ms. BENNETT: She's got us all buggy.

At this point in observation Ms. Bennett and Ms. Donner were mobile and could leave the company of severely impaired patients such as Ms. Zelkan. Others were forced by immobility to remain in the same area. The reaction of Ms. McMurray, one such patient, was considerably more negative.

Ms. ZELKAN: (to Ms. McMurray) Nurse, honey. Please give me that blanket.
Ms. MCMURRAY: No!
Ms. ZELKAN: No?
Ms. MCMURRAY: No!
Ms. ZELKAN: Why? My mother is coming.
Ms. MCMURRAY: No!
Ms. ZELKAN: Do you have an extra fork?
Ms. MCMURRAY: No!
Ms. ZELKAN: Nurse, can you get me my napkin?
Ms. MCMURRAY: No!
Ms. ZELKAN: Why not?
Ms. MCMURRAY: You don't need it!
Ms. ZELKAN: Oh, yes I do! Don't tell me what I need! (emphatically)
Ms. MCMURRAY: No!
Observation: *Ms. McMurray turns her back to Ms. Zelkan. She looks bored and disgusted.*

Indeed, there were some examples that suggest a sort of norm among intact patients to separate themselves from the demented patients. In the following instance, Ms. Bennett (a modestly impaired long-time patient) tries to dissuade a new patient from responding to a severely impaired patient.

> Note: *Fourth-floor television lounge.*
> Ms. Mitnick: Ugh, ugh, ugh.
> Observation: *Ms. Mitnick begins beating rhythmically on the wheelchair table. She is using her fist.*
> Ms. Bennett: Don't go over there. She doesn't need you.
> Mrs. Ruth: What do you want?
> Observation: *Mrs. Ruth walks up to Ms. Mitnick.*
> Ms. Bennett: No, Mrs. Ruth.
> Observation: *Ms. Mitnick begins shaking her tray.*
> Mrs. Ruth: Don't do that.
> Ms. Mitnick: Ugh, ugh, ugh. (shaking the desk)

Even attempts by intact patients to learn what impaired patients wanted in order to assist them were generally not successful. Below, Ms. Kosak observes that a new patient sitting at her table is not eating and tries to intervene.

> Note: *Mrs. Ruth is not eating.*
> Ms. Kosak: Do you need some help with your milk?
> Mrs. Ruth: Some help with the milk?
> Ms. Kosak: Can you open your milk? (louder)
> Mrs. Ruth: I can't open it.
> Observation: *Ms. Kosak opens her milk.*
> Mrs. Ruth: Thank you. Did you get any orange juice?
> Ms. Kosak: Yes.
> Observation: *Mrs. Ruth continues to sit there, neither eating nor drinking.*
> Ms. Kosak: Do you want your milk in a glass?
> Mrs. Ruth: Well . . . I don't know.
> Observation: *Ms. Kosak looks exasperated and appears to give up.*

Attempts by intact patients to support the initiation of activity by impaired patients was infrequent; their attempts to actually assist impaired patients in initiating activity were even more infrequent and, as seen above, generally not too successful.

One would expect the most from the relationships between cognitively intact patients, and while there were few patients on the ward who were not somewhat cognitively compromised, it was indeed here where we saw the most basis for support for autonomy. For example, Ms. Hofsky often took Ms. Kosak back up to the fourth floor from the dining hall. This allowed Ms. Kosak to decide when she wanted to leave after the mealtime was over, rather than having to wait in line for staff to move her.

In another instance we noted, Ms. Hofsky took Ms. Graves down to the patient accounts office. It was through this office that patients received small amounts of cash from a fund kept for each. Without Ms. Hofsky's assistance, Ms. Graves would have had to wait until a volunteer had time to bring her down. That delay in access might have been a day or more.

> Observation: *Meanwhile, Ms. Hofsky rolls Ms. Graves over to the visitor elevator. They were down in the patient accounts office. As they wait by the elevator, Ms. Hofsky explains the patient accounts system to Ms. Graves. She seems to enjoy this.*

In another example, Ms. Baker provides some support for Mrs. Randle's interest in playing cards, implying that she would also be interested in playing.

> Note: *Third-floor television lounge.*
> MRS. RANDLE: Do you ever play cards here?
> MS. BAKER: Well, the Catholics play on Sunday, so we can play on Sunday.
> MRS. RANDLE: Yes.

Over the course of time, a close relationship developed between Mrs. Randle and Ms. Baker. They generally sat in the television lounge together, read together, ate together, and attended activities together. This relationship, however, appeared to be the only close, supportive one between intact patients on the mixed care unit.

There were two similar relationships on the skilled unit: between Ms. Gartner and Ms. Castra, and between Ms. Hofsky and Ms. Lyndon. Ms. Lyndon, however, was bedfast and incapable of verbal communication. Unable for the most part to communicate with her roommate, Ms. Lyndon primarily just listened to Ms. Hofsky talk to her and allowed Ms. Hofsky to feed her.

Ms. Gartner and Ms. Castra, on the other hand, were not significantly cognitively impaired. They spent much of their time sitting together in the hallway, talking and occasionally laughing about what they saw go on about them. Excerpts from observation indicate a warm, supportive relationship.

> Observation: *Ms. Gartner and Ms. Castra are best buddies. [They have both had strokes and] consequently, it is quite difficult to understand [them but they] can understand each other quite well. It is common to see them sitting together—wheelchair to wheelchair—in the hallway talking and laughing. . . . Occasionally, Ms. Gartner would refer to Ms. Castra as "Buttercup." This seemed to be some sort of running joke between them.*

Although examples indicative of supportive relationships do not provide evidence of support for specific behaviors, they do suggest that the climate for such support does exist to a limited degree among intact patients.

On the other hand, there are several examples in which patients discouraged other patients from undertaking activities counter to the institutional routine.

> MS. BENNETT: I want to go to bed.
> MS. FLORENCE: You can't go to bed. You just ate dinner.

Ms. Bennett frequently requested to go to bed early, and was rarely allowed by staff to do so. Ms. Florence's comment thus served to support the legitimacy of the institutional patterns.

Ms. Baker's and Mrs. Randle's criticism of Ms. Viancia reflected a tendency of some patients to support the views of the staff.

> Note: *Ms. Baker and Mrs. Randle are talking in the third-floor lounge.*
> MRS. RANDLE: Ms. Viancia is one. If the doctor says she should have something to drink, before she'd be out the door, she'd say no. If he said she shouldn't have anything to drink, before she was out the door, she'd have something.
> MS. BAKER: Yeah. Yeah.

Conclusion

There are a variety of factors that mitigate against patient/patient relationships providing a significant social support system for autonomous behavior. The most demented patients seem unlikely to be able to sustain such interactions among themselves and the more cognitively able patients seem disinclined to help, perhaps drawing boundaries that allow them to sustain a self-image as competent individuals.

There is some reason, however, to be optimistic about the possibility of these relationships among the cognitively intact patients. While some such patients sustained no substantial contacts with other patients, some developed close and lasting relationships. In the facility we studied, the cognitively competent patients often seemed lost among the demented. It seems possible that if a facility separated out the cognitively intact or minimally impaired patients from the more impaired that patient/patient support for autonomy might increase.

NOTES

1. We coded 66 requests for assistance, 5 requests for permission, and 131 requests for information. In addition there were 117 nonspecific requests which were mostly from very demented patients.

2. We noted earlier that we had a lot of difficulty observing the behavior of residents because they did not interact much in public. This might seem to argue against this and other comments about the differences between resident-staff and patient-staff interaction. However, the fact is that we spent considerable time with residence staff without seeing the incessant requests that we observed routinely in the intermediate and mixed nursing care settings.

3. The field observations contain 348 different speaking turns of direct interaction between patients.

9

Privacy: Access to Space and Property

When we talk about the right to confidentiality, we are referring to a person's ability to control access by others to several different facets of her world including space, information, and personally meaningful objects. The protection of privacy is directly related to the protection of the sense of autonomous selfhood. Focusing on private information, Rem Edwards notes:

> Such facts lie at the core of our identity as distinctive individuals; and in cherishing and protecting them, we may be either positively evaluating our own well-being and unique individuality or protecting ourselves from certain harms which would befall us if others know things about us that were none of their damned business. Some of these private facts about ourselves are so secret that we will never relate them to anyone. Some of these facts we will relate to a close circle of acquaintances. . . . Still others we will relate to an even wider circle of acquaintances, and there are many facts about ourselves which we will relate to anyone who wants to know. . . (Edwards 1988).

The connection to the sense of an autonomous self equally involves other facets of privacy including restriction on access to specific spaces and objects. Privacy often involves a restriction that is claimed as an individual or group right, and it restricts access to something that is socially defined as uniquely tied to a particular person or group.

Every group or institution has some rules that organize access to space, information, and physical objects and determine the extent of individuals' privacy rights. Thus, for example, a research group will have rules that regulate access to research files, restricting it to those involved in the project. Likewise hospitals have visiting hours that restrict outsiders' access to hospital floors and patients who inhabit them during certain periods. Informal family rules may restrict the children's access to the parents' bedrooms and, in turn, as they grow older, children may attempt to restrict access to their rooms.

More generally, in our society, we protect individuals' rights to restrict access to information, personal objects, and spaces. This right is differentially protected depending on our relationship to the person who wishes access. The Fourth Amendment of the Constitution, for example, places severe restrictions on the access of an agent of the state to our homes and, somewhat less so, to our automobiles and bodies when they inhabit public spaces.[1] On the other hand, spouses are allowed into many of our most private spaces and often are told many of our deepest secrets.

It is the relationship of the notion of privacy to the individual's core sense of self that makes it of such interest in the study of autonomy. Allowing persons some control over personal information is important to developing a sense of personal identity. Moreover, highly personal information about ourselves can affect our lives in significant ways, and we typically wish to have control over how this information is distributed and to whom. A lack of privacy can have a negative impact on one's autonomy. As Goffman (1961) has pointed out, total institutions, such as army camps and monasteries, routinely do not grant privacy to inmates in even the most intimate of activities. In doing so they break down some of the individuality of the inmates which is thought to interfere with the achievement of the goals of the organization. Thus, aside from being a matter of substantial importance in itself, by observing the ways in which the institution allocates privacy rights we can learn something about how the long-term care facility influences individual autonomy.

Spatial Rights

One of the more important components of privacy is the ability to control other's entry into "private" spaces. This ability to control one's space is particularly important in nursing homes. Patient's rooms are their *de facto* homes, the place where they keep their most prized and intimate possessions. These rooms may also be the only places in the institution to which patients can go to get away from others. Nursing home patients are usually physically unable to go outside the institution to find "private" spaces. They must depend on institutional policies that delineate and protect areas for their privacy.

In order to discuss the ways in which spatial rights were allocated we need to review briefly the physical layout of the nursing care units. Both the intermediate and mixed skilled and intermediate floors resembled hospital units; each consisted of long hallways opening into small rooms on both sides, with a staff station situated midway down the hall. A handrail ran down both sides of these hallways, providing the means by which ambulatory but unsteady patients could navigate. The staff station, which was separated from the hallway by a high counter, contained patient records and a locked medications cabinet, with the records and a variety of medical supplies, work schedules, and posted notices in plain view. Adjacent to this area was a small staff lounge, where line staff spent their free time. The majority of patient rooms were designed for double occupancy, with two single rooms each on the skilled and intermediate floors.

Areas available to patients included their rooms and two television lounges per unit. Lounges were located at opposite ends of the hallway. The larger lounge on each unit was capable of accommodating approximately twenty people, and was generally filled with patients restrained in wheelchairs and geri-chairs. The small lounge on each unit could hold roughly ten people, and was generally empty when not being used by families during visits.

The furnishings of each patient room also resembled what one would expect to see in a hospital. A double room typically contained a hospital-issue bed, a nightstand, and a small rolling table for each occupant, with a shared dresser, cupboard, and bathroom. Single rooms contained a second dresser or bookcase and occasionally an easy chair. The furniture was supplied by the nursing home and was standard hospital stock. Thus admission to the nursing home required patients to give up many of their personal possessions and much of their individuality.

Only minimal efforts were taken to protect patients' privacy once admitted to the nursing home. Each double room contained a curtain suspended between the two beds, which was often pulled by staff to allow patients privacy during dressing and other ADLs. However, the privacy afforded patients by this curtain was limited; sounds and smells were not contained, and movement could be clearly seen. Moreover, the doors to both single and double patient rooms were left open during the day and night, allowing staff—as well as other patients and visitors—to observe patients from the hallway. Pulling the curtain across in a double room provided little privacy for patients who lived on the hallway side of the room.

> Note: *Ms. Kosak occupied the bed nearest the hallway.*
> Observation: *As I walk down the hall, I can see Ms. Kosak. She is sitting on a portable commode right inside her room.*

The few exceptions to the open-door policy occurred when patients were acutely ill or staff were performing certain medical tasks. For example, the door to Mr. Maginn's room was kept closed from the time he returned from the hospital until he died from gangrene a few weeks later. Likewise, room doors were generally closed when staff were reinserting naso-gastric tubes or performing other substantial medical procedures.

It is not entirely clear why room doors routinely remained open. It might be assumed that this policy was designed so that staff could monitor patients' conditions in an attempt to prevent possible injury. This is the explanation that is typically given in hospitals for leaving patient's doors open. However, it is hard to see why this rule should not apply to the most seriously ill patients.[2] Moreover, most nursing home patients are not acutely ill and are at fairly low risk of self injury. In general, we are inclined to view the general policy as one more indicator of the ways in which the institution reflected its medical roots.

Since there were no barriers to their doing so, it is not surprising that staff generally entered patients' rooms without warning. Line staff, in particular, appeared to enter occupied rooms at their discretion; we did not observe any instances in which these staff either knocked on the open doors or called out prior to entering patients' rooms.

In one instance, however, an aide did apologize after entering a patient's room while the patient and observer were talking.

> Note: *The observer and Ms. Kosak are sitting in a room shared by Ms. Kosak and Ms. Mitnick.*
> Observation: *We are interrupted by an unidentified aide. She rolls Ms. Mitnick into the room.*
> UNIDENTIFIED AIDE: (to observer) Sorry to barge in like that. I thought you were done. Or went back to the lounge.
> MS. KOSAK: You wanna bring her in now? (referring to Ms. Mitnick)
> AIDE: That's what they tell me.

The aide's apology for "barging in" was atypical. The apology was apparently directed to the observer, and not to Ms. Kosak. Apparently, the observer, as a professional, was accorded some privacy rights that patients were not. This is the only instance we observed in which staff apologized for an intrusion.

Sometimes patients found staff intrusions to be acutely embarrassing. For example:

> US–15: One night I was putting her (Ms. Owen) back (into bed from the bathroom), and I was halfway getting her into bed. Her back end was sticking out, and (a male aide) came in the door. . . . She just did a real quick turn around with her head, and she said, "Oh, get out of here!" I went and stood in front of her to kind of cover her up.

However, such embarrassment seems to have been unusual. Some cognitively impaired patients may not have been alert enough to understand their rights were being violated. Among the relatively few cognitively intact patients, there was some frustration about their lack of privacy. However, most of this frustration appeared to center on their being forced to share rooms. Their anger was thus focused on Medicare reimbursement policies, which specified that patients must share rooms. One cognitively intact patient on Medicare described for us her lack of privacy and her attempts to cope with having to share her room with a series of impaired roommates.

> OBSERVER: Your roommate, Ms. Mitnick, seems to be pretty much out of it most of the time.
> MS. KOSAK: Yeah, she is. She's disoriented and a little nasty sometimes. She scratches people and pinches people.
> OBSERVER: Do you have any trouble getting along with her?
> MS. KOSAK: She doesn't bother me. I went past her one day and she scratched me. But I never particularly bother with her. I just get them.
> OBSERVER: You mean the roommates that you get?
> MS. KOSAK: Oh, yes.
> OBSERVER: What kind of roommates have you had?
> MS. KOSAK: I have had quite a few. They're kind of bad. Some of them are. . . .
> OBSERVER: The ones that are bad . . . what do you mean by bad?
> MS. KOSAK: Difficult to get along with, like Ms. Mitnick.
> OBSERVER: Do you have any choice about who you have for a roommate?
> MS. KOSAK: No. Personally, I'd rather not have anybody.
> OBSERVER: You'd like a private room?
> MS. KOSAK: Yes. But our contract stipulates (reference to Medicare reimbursement) . . . the only thing to do is try to be active as much as I can.
> OBSERVER: By active, you mean outside the room?
> MS. KOSAK: Outside the facility. Outside the room. Just wherever I can.

That this, rather than staff intrusions, was the focus of complaints from patients reflects the pervasiveness of the expectations about the staff role.

The lack of privacy in the rooms was made more difficult by the fact that there were no areas within the facility where patients could go to be alone. At best there were communal areas such as the study lounge and the chapel. The amount of privacy one could get by going to these areas, however, was limited by the fact that they were seldom occupied by only one person. Upper staff were aware that there was little private space available to patients.

> OBSERVER: I was just trying to imagine being in a place like this. There really is no place for privacy, or at least one that is readily available.
> NURSING SUPERVISOR: I think that's the thing that would destroy me, too. I'm a very personal person, and it would be really rough to not have an hour when there was nobody there to bother me. Even if you pick up and go somewhere else, there's no guarantee that someone will not intrude on your space.

While most line staff did not seem to see their actions (eg, entering rooms without knocking) as problematic, upper staff appeared concerned. However, they generally saw such intrusions as inherent in the system and unchangeable.

Our interviews with, and observations of, family members reflected little concern about patients' privacy within the nursing home context. Their concern about space was limited to concern about specific rooming situations. The comments that did surface were made primarily in the context of admissions tours. In the following example, for instance, the daughter of a potential patient expresses her preference that her father be in a private room or share his room with another cognitively intact individual. The issue is raised only once during the tour, and there is no evidence that the family attempted to modify his room assignment after he was admitted.

> DAUGHTER: I was wondering . . . would he be put in with someone?
> UPPER STAFF–05: We have no private rooms [available].
> DAUGHTER: We (daughter and wife) were wondering if . . . possibly . . . if he could be put in with someone who was clear-headed?
> US–05: We try to match up people as best we can. Sometimes it's pretty hard.
> WIFE: There's nothing wrong with his mind.

> US–05: Well, it would be hard for me to promise the exact room situation right now. . . .[3]

Another way in which staff ignored patient's privacy was their entry into unoccupied patient rooms. In general patients remained unaware of staff entry into their rooms. Such events occurred most frequently during admissions tours given for families. However, admissions tours did not always lead to such entries.

> Note: *Admissions tour.*
> Observation: . . . *then [an upper staff member] leads them down the hallway.*
> US–05: And here is a private room.
> Observation: *She gestures to room 6040. The two women (family members) walk toward it.*
> US–05: We're not going to be able to go in there. We can't go in without his (patient's) permission.

More typically staff were not so hesitant, especially when the patients being considered for admission were likely to be admitted.[4] For instance, it is interesting that the same staff member described above was willing to violate her own rule when it was likely that the patient would be admitted:

> Note: *Discussion with the family and a pre-tour financial check have indicated that the patient in question was likely to be admitted.*
> Observation: *We (upper staff, observer, family members) walk down the hallway. The admissions coordinator points out several rooms, describing their features in detail. Then we walk down to the far television lounge. Following that, US–05 leads the two men into room 6020.*
> US–05: This lady isn't here. We really should ask her permission first before coming in, but I don't think she would care anyway.
> Observation: *[We enter.] US–05 points out . . . features of the room, stressing the call button. Then we go up the hallway.*

Staff views regarding patients' right to privacy can be contrasted with the value they placed on their ability to maintain a private area for themselves. The door to the staff lounge was generally shut. Although staff was not systematically excluded from any space, patients were generally forbidden to enter either the staff station or adjacent lounge area. The pay telephones for both the intermediate and skilled units were located in these lounges and patients were sometimes allowed to use those phones, but only with explicit staff permission. Otherwise, these were absolutely off-limits and patient attempts to enter were reacted to quite negatively.

Privacy of Possessions

There was one other circumstance in which staff entered patients' rooms without their consent, indeed, sometimes against their expressed wishes:

> Observation: *We (nurse, aide, and observer) walked down the hallway, and into room 4024. It is Ms. Donner's room.*
> N–01: I'm trying to clean this lady's room. She's like a little hermit. She doesn't want us to move anything. So you've got to sneak in here while she's gone.
> Observation: *A–02 and N–01 move around the room, vacuuming and dusting.*
> N–01: Soon she'll have some friends in here. Little mice and everything. (laughs)
> A–02: Oh, my god.
> OBSERVATION: *N–01 finds a stash of food (cookies, etc.) in the corner. She carries it into the bathroom and dumps it into the wastebasket. I can hear the sound of singing from the lounge. A–02 begins to vacuum again, while N–01 moves furniture out of the way for her.*

Staff regularly entered Ms. Donner's room against her wishes in order to vacuum. In the process of cleaning they sometimes discarded things that were of little monetary value but had some value to her. In doing so they violated her privacy (ie, her claim to have special access and control over them). In this instance the staff judged that sanitation and safety were more important than any such claims.

While the majority of privacy issues concerned space, the issue of personal property was also relevant. In the following example, a resident monitor tells a nurse about a situation in which the institutionalized sister of a deceased patient recognized her sister's clothing being worn by another patient:

> MONITOR: (paraphrased discussion) When the deceased patient's sister saw another patient wearing her sister's clothing, she became upset. . . . When she saw someone else wearing the clothes she said, "But you have to give them back. She will be cold. Someone else can't have her clothes. She needs them in order to be warm."

The staff's appropriation and distribution of the deceased patient's clothing was probably motivated by a desire to provide clothing for a needy patient. However, the disposing of deceased individual's personal possessions within our culture is a task generally reserved for family, and frequently functions to help persons grieve. In appropriating the deceased patient's belongings, staff provided needed clothing for another patient but took away from the patient's sister the ability to perform a culturally accepted ritual. Once again the privacy issues were subordinated to other legitimate concerns.

Information Privacy

Structuring the nursing home like a hospital resulted in patients' privacy being violated in another way. Confidentiality in the nursing home was nonexistent. Just as in a hospital (Siegler 1982), staff were privy to all information about all patients. It was not uncommon for a staff member who was caring for a patient to tell a staff member who was not caring for the patient fairly sensitive information about that patient. Moreover this information was sometimes discussed in relatively public areas in which others could overhear. Often this information was more salient as gossip than as medical information the staff needed to know to care for the patient. In one instance a physician passed on to the staff observations he made during a patient's physical examination:

> Note: *An upper staff member is responding to the observer's question about Mr. Scheff's reluctance to bathe.*
> US–03: . . . maybe he didn't like females bathing him. I don't know of any guys up there (another floor) doing it for him. . . . Dr X thought it was more of a sexual thing. He told some of the nurses, from just examining him, that his penis was real small. I guess his testicles were real small too. Maybe he didn't want to have anybody see it.

Bodily Privacy

We also saw a number of instances of what might be called "violations of bodily privacy." These actions, which usually occurred against the patient's expressed wishes, have special importance for our study of autonomy. Although it can be argued that physical restraint is one such instance, our discussion here will be limited to issues concerning medical tasks and the performance of ADLs (eg, eating, bathing, toileting), since we discuss physical restraints in Chapter 10.

> Observation: *As I step off the elevator, I see N–03 heading down the hallway, carrying a small plastic cup with some kind of medication in it. She comes up to Mrs. Graves from behind, and grabs the front of her hair with her left hand. She pulls Mrs. Graves' head back and quickly pours the medication into her mouth. Mrs. Graves looks like she doesn't know what has happened to her. Part of the medication runs back out her mouth.*

This approach, although not frequent, was used periodically with patients considered uncooperative. Mrs. Graves, a cognitively intact cerebral palsy patient, often bothered staff with aggressive demands and was thus considered a problem patient by some staff, especially N–03. This method allowed her to quickly administer the medication to Mrs. Graves while negating the possibility of refusal or another request.

This approach was more often used with impaired patients who sometimes seemed unaware that they were being given medication.

> Observation: *Ms. Davies (a nurse) goes up to the kitchenette and comes back with a small container of ice cream. She crushes up some pills and stirs them in the ice cream. She walks to Ms. Stark, who is sitting in her geri-chair in the hallway.*
> Ms. Davies: Ms. Stark, your ice cream.
> Observation: *There is no response from the patient. She appears to be asleep.*
> Ms. Davies: Ms. Stark. (louder) Now you're waking up.
> Observation: *Ms. Davies pushes Ms. Stark's head back with her left hand, and puts a tongue depressor with ice cream and pills on it into her mouth. The patient swallows.*

A somewhat different issue of bodily privacy was the staff's practice of routinely performing medical procedures such as cleaning leg ulcers, and changing IV bottles and feeding tubes in public areas such as the TV lounge. In fact, most procedures (excluding naso-gatric tubes) were done wherever the patients were when the staff found them.[5] Only when family was present were most procedures—even giving eye drops—conducted in patients' rooms.

It should be clear that privacy of space, information, possessions, or body, was not a norm stressed in the nursing home. Three factors seemed to make staff comfortable with substantial limitations on patients' privacy. First, the medical model from which the institution derives much of its identity and legitimacy accepts such features as routine. Second, staff tends to see the loss of patient privacy as appropriate when such other values as sanitation and good relations with the patients' relatives are enhanced. Finally, one gets the sense that staff felt more comfortable invading patient's privacy because many of them were demented and not aware of what was happening to them. This combined with the fact that most patients did not complain about their privacy being violated may have led staff to be comfortable with their behavior.

Residential Units

The residential living quarters were noticeably different from the patient units. Although each of the three floors consisted of a hallway with small rooms set on both sides, the hallways were carpeted and decorated with pictures. There were no formal staff stations, but rather one small office on each floor where staff met at shift changes. This staff area was accessible to residents, and they typically wandered in and out of this area. The atmosphere on this unit was closer to that of a hotel or apartment house than a hospital.

All rooms on the residential units were designed for single occupancy, although some residents did share a bath. The rooms were approximately the same size as those on the patient units, but recently had been remodeled and contained no hospital-issue furniture. Residents were encouraged to bring their own furniture and, consequently, there was little similarity between rooms.

The doors to residents' rooms were kept shut most of the time. When residents were off the unit, their doors were locked; while they were on the unit, doors were unlocked, but closed. Each resident carried a room key, while resident monitors possessed master keys. The most frequent exception to closed doors occurred at night; some residents wanted their doors left ajar so that staff could hear them if they called out.

Staff generally knocked on residents' doors before entering, but they rarely waited for a response before entering the room.

> Observation: *We (observer and staff) go into Ms. Kelly's room. Ms. Smith (a resident nurse) knocks before she enters, and then pushes the door open. Ms. Kelly is stretched out on her bed, covered with an*

> *afghan and fast asleep. We go on down to Kathryn's room. Ms. Smith knocks and then goes in. Kathryn talks to us while trying to put hair-pins in her hair.*

One monitor, in particular, had quick entry down to an art form.

> Observation: *She (monitor) insisted on showing me six of the (residents') rooms. She had a master key that opened all the doors. Before knocking on the doors, she would put the key into the lock. Then, before the residents had time to respond . . . , Ms. Lee turned the lock and was in the room.*

Occasionally, this resulted in what most people would perceive as embarrassing situations.

> Observation: *She (resident monitor) walked into Ms. Walters' room. The door was ajar. The light was on and the radio was playing loudly. Ms. Walters was sitting in the bathroom (on the commode). Ms. Baker walked into the bathroom and they had a conversation.*

The residents, however, did not seem to object to staff entry into their rooms without permission, even when it resulted in situations such as the one above. Instead, most seemed pleased to have someone with whom to talk. As seen in Chapter 5, residential staff spoke of residents as part of their family, and reported working to promote family-type relationships. It is possible to interpret resident-staff behavior concerning room entry within that framework. Whether such an interpretation is justified is difficult to assess.

Whereas staff were unchallenged in suspending typical rules of privacy, this privilege did not extend to other residents.

> MRS. REED: You know that little girl I was sitting with out there?
> OBSERVER: Yes.
> Observation: *She must be referring to Ms. Zabotnik.*
> MRS. REED: Well, she just follows me wherever I go. I just can't get rid of her. Wherever I go, she's there. (pause) You know, I caught her standing outside of my door the other day. I was sitting in here (room) talking on the phone and she was standing outside my door, listening.

> I told her not to do that. I really laid into her. (emphatically) I just won't put up with that.

While it is possible that residents simply differentiated between staff and other residents as family and outsiders, respectively, and tolerated invasions of privacy by "family" but not outsiders, other plausible explanations exist. Although theoretically capable of independent living, many residents were actually impaired, both physically and cognitively, and thus dependent on staff for considerable help with ADLs. These residents remained in the residence primarily due to the efforts of resident monitors, who picked up the slack for residents unable to care for themselves. It is possible, then, that some residents tolerated violations of their privacy by staff out of fear that if they objected monitors might withhold the assistance they needed to remain in an independent living setting. This could explain the absence of objections by residents to violations of privacy by staff, but their intolerance of the same actions by other residents. We have, unfortunately, no data to settle this question.

There were few examples of privacy violations on these units. The most frequent infraction related to information. As in the nursing home, confidentiality was often not honored. Often monitors found out information from families that the resident had not told them, in particular about the resident's disposal of property outside the facility. Only a handful of examples of violation of personal possessions were identified, and we saw no evidence of violations of the body.

> Observation: *Interview with Ms. Black.*
> MS. BLACK: OK, Ms. Martin has a bladder problem. She normally tends to herself, but when she has an accident she just gets very embarrassed and upset and. . . .
> OBSERVER: Is it fairly common for her?
> MS. BLACK: Yes, it is. She . . . up until a couple of months ago . . . she was doctoring herself. She'd have Kaopectate over there, and Milk of Magnesia. And she was taking them at the wrong time. So we just went in and kind of confiscated all that.

In general, residents were afforded greater privacy than patients. The most noticeable difference was the residents' option to keep their room doors locked or at least closed. This allowance, however, was not without limits; staff had pass keys which they used to enter occupied as well as unoccupied rooms at their discretion.

Conclusion

We have tried to emphasize that, in these settings, the ability to act as autonomous agents is often dependent on an individual's perception of herself as independent and in control. Respect for privacy is, among other things, one of the ways in which we symbolize our acknowledgement that the person is an autonomous agent who is in control of her life. This respect can be shown by respecting a person's ability to control information, or by respecting their possessions. However, probably the most important way one respects another's privacy is by allowing them a socially defined space into which others cannot go without their permission. In the wider society, most working and middle class adults have a space to call their own—their home. The ability to put a locked door between themselves and the rest of the world symbolizes, in a dramatic way, that the space is theirs. If one wishes to enter that space one must knock on the door and wait to be permitted entrance. The residential side, while hardly total privacy, made an effort to ensure the residents some privacy. The door was shut and the lock was there. In the nursing units, however, rooms were shared, doors were open, and almost anyone could obtain unrestricted access to patients' space. Few metaphors seemed to capture the different levels of institutional support for autonomy as well as the ways in which access to patients' and residents' rooms was handled.

NOTES

1. There is, of course, an ongoing debate about the extent of such restrictions on personal privacy rights. In *Roe* vs *Wade* the US Supreme Court seemed to create a wide area of rights to privacy. In recent years however this has been somewhat restricted and there is considerable feeling in "conservative" circles that it should be abolished.

2. In fact, in the hospital setting access to more seriously ill patients is maximized, ie, they are placed closer to the nursing station and doors are left open at all times. The only case where this is not true in a hospital is where the patient is clearly going to die and has requested that life-sustaining treatment be foregone. In this situation, which may be more analogous to Mr. Maginn's case, the doors are usually kept shut.

3. It is likely that the staff member's reluctance to commit herself was dictated partly by the small number of cognitively intact individuals on the unit and partly by the limits of her role responsibilities, which left the pairing of roommates to other staff.

4. The shortest tours, and those least likely to include patients' rooms, were generally given to families whose patients were, for any of a variety of reasons, unlikely to be admitted.

5. Watching these more complicated procedures take place in the halls emphasized the medical nature of the units.

10

Physical Redirection and Restraint

There are few issues more directly relevant to autonomy in long-term care than staff's use of physical force and restraint. Much of our concern about autonomy for the elderly in long-term care is based on our image of the elderly woman tied up by those who "care for her." Of course, as we have tried to show here, the loss of autonomy in nursing care institutions is not primarily a problem of physical force. On the contrary, there are a variety of subtle ways in which individual agency is undercut and constrained in the nursing home setting. However, the use of force to control an elderly individual's intentional action remains a major concern. While we have already discussed briefly some of these issues in Chapter 4, the topic requires a more detailed discussion.

In assessing the impact of these behaviors on patients' lives, we immediately run into both a methodological problem and an evaluative one. The methodological problem is that the impact of the staff's use of force presumably carries over into many other behaviors in which force is not used. The implicit or explicit threat of force may have a much greater influence on patient behavior than the few instances in which force is actually used. Since force was most often used on demented patients who have great difficulty recounting their motives, it is difficult to assess the impact of threats on their behavior.

The evaluative problem is even more difficult. The problem is that it is simply too glib to take a moral position that helping professionals and paraprofessionals should not use force to modify the behavior of those whom they are helping. This position forgets that all of these interactions take place in real life organizations. All organizations have power structures that are necessary to accomplish their goals and all power, ultimately, must rest on some sort of base of force (Mosca, 1939). Put more simply, the use or threat of power is a uniform feature of all social organizations.

It is also clearly true that different organizations use more or less force to accomplish their goals.[1] To some degree this is dictated by the task. Nursing homes clearly cannot use the complex set of symbolic appeals that, for example, an elite university might use to gain the cooperation of its faculty. For some demented patients there is considerable question about whether a more sophisticated sanctioning system would be useful in gaining their cooperation.

In spite of these difficulties, this chapter will try to describe the various ways in which physical force was used to gain patient cooperation in hopes of providing an empirical context within which a normative evaluation would be possible. We will begin by describing what we came to call "physical redirection," ie, physical acts on the part of staff that were designed to affect the patients' immediate short-term behavior.[2]

Physical Redirection

Many of the line staff's attempts at redirection consisted of attempts to prevent patient injuries.

> Observation: *Ms. Linley (an aide) takes Ms. Kramer's tray off the cart and sets it on the coffee table beside her. She begins cutting up the food. Ms. Kramer reaches for the food.*
> Ms. Linley: Ms. Kramer, don't touch that. It's hot.
> Ms. Kramer: Don't touch it? (sounds puzzled)
> Ms. Linley: That's right. Don't touch it.
> Observation: *Ms. Kramer pulls her hand back. Then she reaches for the tray again.*
> Ms. Linley: No, no, no, no, no, no, no!
> Observation: *Ms. Linley takes Ms. Kramer's hand from the coffee cup and puts it back over on her lap.*
> Ms. Linley: It's hot, Ms. Kramer.
> Observation: *Ms. Linley finishes cutting up Ms. Kramer's food and puts a plate of it on Ms. Kramer's wheelchair desk. Ms. Kramer begins to eat with her hands.*

Although redirection was used primarily with severely impaired patients, less impaired patients were also redirected by staff. While only mildly impaired, Mr. Friedman had a history of trying to ignore the physical limitations imposed by his stroke.

> Observation: *Ms. Baker comes down the hallway to the TV lounge.*
> Ms. Baker: (Mr. Friedman) You have a call. It's your daughter.
> Mr. Friedman: Oh . . . (several sentences in Yiddish)
> Ms. Baker: What's wrong?
> Observation: *Ms. Baker sounds agitated.*
> Mr. Friedman: You don't understand . . . (more Yiddish)
> Note: *Mr. Friedman and his daughter are having a running battle over the management of his finances. (Mr. Friedman leans forward as if to get up.)*
> Ms. Baker: Sit back. Sit back.
> Observation: *Ms. Baker sounds impatient. She reaches forward and pushes Mr. Friedman back into his wheelchair.*
> Ms. Baker: You're going to fall out of there.

In these cases, physical redirection was not used to prevent patients from attaining their goals. Instead, staff set limits that allowed patients to reach their goals and decreased the probability of injury. For example, Mr. Friedman was not restricted from talking with his daughter on the phone. Instead, the aide encouraged him to roll his wheelchair down the hallway to the staff telephone rather than walk there.

Although some instances of physical redirection reflected a physical safety norm, others were used to insure patient compliance with routine institutional norms. Below, for example, Ms. Donner is reminded that patients are required to remain at their tables while eating their meals.

> Observation: *Ms. Donner has rolled her wheelchair back from the table. . . . Occasionally she drinks some juice from the container she holds in her hand. One of the dietary aides moves over to her.*
> Aide: Move up to the table to finish your juice, Ms. Donner.
> Observation: *The aide does not wait for Ms. Donner to move herself. Instead, she rolls her back up to the table. Ms. Donner, as usual, looks dazed.*

While in some ways this is a trivial example of physical redirection since a minimal level of force was used, it clearly shows how physical redirection was used to maintain the system's informal rules. The rule concerning staying at the table until the meal time ended did not protect patients. It was simply one of the many rules the institution had to regulate everyday behavior. While in this instance it probably could have been enforced by discussing it with the patient, in other instances such rules could only be enforced through the use of threats or physical force.

Mr. McLaughlin, for example, was restricted from his room during the day and often could be kept out only by force.

> Note: *The patient is sitting in his wheelchair outside his room door. He is trying to get the door open. I am watching him from several feet away.*
> Ms. Biggs (a nurse, speaking to the observer): He can't go in there. (referring to the patient's room) Mr. McLaughlin, you're not going in there.
> Observation: *He points to his room door.*
> Ms. Biggs: No, Mr. McLaughlin.
> Observation: *He yells some gibberish.*
> Ms. Biggs: No!
> Observation: *She pulls his room door [completely] shut. In response, he kicks at the closed door with his right foot.*
> Ms. Biggs: (to me) If we let him in there he tries to get into the bed. The last time we let him in the room he almost made it into bed while still strapped in his geri-chair.
> Observation: *He continues to yell. Then he stops yelling and begins drooling. She rolls him [around] to sit in front of the closed door.*

While Ms. Biggs justified the use of force in terms of the patient's physical safety, this was a bit disingenuous; numerous comments by staff indicated that they did not want patients to nap during the day because it meant that they would be up at night. This, in turn, was a problem because the institution, like most nursing facilities, had fewer staff at night. Staff, therefore, worked hard to minimize the amount of work that needed to be done during the night shift. While Ms. Biggs's concern for protecting the patient's safety undoubtedly was genuine, it was clearly secondary. The dangerous behavior, his attempt to get into bed while still in a geri-chair, could have been prevented by simply helping him into his bed. Here, and elsewhere, given patients' cognitive impairment and the techniques of behavioral control with which the line staff was familiar, physical force was a necessary means for accomplishing the organization's rules and policies.[3]

Staff frustration with patients sometimes led to the use of threats or physical force. As we noted elsewhere, staff experienced considerable frustration in interacting with cognitively impaired patients, particularly those patients who were uncooperative. This frustration generally did not lead to anything more serious than an occasional threat.

> Observation: *Mr. Friedman does not look up at me, but he does make a noise. I don't know whether he's trying to talk to me or not. . . . Ms. Kennedy (an aide) comes out of a patient's room. Mr. Friedman grunts at her.*
> Ms. Kennedy: (apparently she can understand him) You know you can't do that. If you don't stop that, I'm going to beat you!
> Observation: *Ms. Marshall (an aide) comes down the hallway pushing an empty wheelchair. [We talked about the research project.] She told me that "to deal with some patients you just have to scream at them."*

However, on a few occasions things got more serious.

> Observation: *As we talked I heard raised voices from the third-floor lounge area. I saw Nurse Sprye and Mr. Viancia struggling with each other. Ms. Sprye was trying to force Mr. Viancia up from his wheelchair and into a geri-chair. Mr. Viancia was . . . resisting. Ms. Sprye was pulling Mr. Viancia forward by his shoulders. Mr. Viancia was swinging at Ms. Sprye's head. Finally, the nurse yanked the patient forward, spun him around, and threw him into the geri-chair. . . . Mr. Viancia kept swinging at the nurse's head as the nurse fastened the geri-chair into place.*

These behaviors only serve to re-emphasize the problems that line staff experienced in trying both to ensure patient safety and maintain institutional order. In the absence of other effective techniques, it is not surprising that staff sometimes resorted to threats or physical redirection in order to ensure patient compliance.

Restraints

Perhaps the best introduction to the topic of physical restraints was provided by one of the upper staff who said: "If you talk about an autonomy issue, the 'frailty, falling, clapped in a geri-chair syndrome' is probably, in a nursing facility, the key autonomy issue."[4]

Almost without exception, restraints were used with cognitively impaired patients. Sometimes physical restraints were employed after other attempts at redirection had failed. More often, however, physical restraints appeared to be staff's first response to a problem. Their use was sometimes prompted by accidents or near accidents. Mr. Friedman is the patient described above as being redirected by an aide in an effort to keep him from falling.

> Observation: *Nurse Biggs walks [another staff member] down to Mr. Friedman's room. I follow.*
> OBSERVER: What happened?
> MS. BAKER (an aide): He fell out of his chair. We found him on the floor.
> OBSERVER: Did he hurt himself?
> MS. BAKER: No. But we figured we'd better restrain him so he couldn't do it again.

At other times, however, restraints were used prior to the patient's having had an accident. Staff used restraints in what they considered potentially troublesome situations to prevent accidents. In the example below, staff anticipated difficulty with a patient whose sedation was being reduced.

> Note: *Staff report.*
> NURSE: Mr. McLaughlin had a change in his medication after he was seen by the doctor. He now gets Haldol . . . only . . . uh, the b.i.d. was cut. He (doctor) does not want a PRN order at this time. The family called the doctor and said that, uh . . . Pt–11 was oversedated. He was drooling and a lot of the time he's been lethargic. He was noisy at intervals last night. He has the posey around him, but it is not tied to the bed. It was until about 4 AM He was fussing about it so I did untie it and it has remained that way.

The response of patients to such limitations of their mobility varied. Newly admitted patients, in particular, tended to voice strong objections.

> Observation: *Mr. Borza is lying in the lounge, strapped down on a type of gurney. He is a very tall, heavy white male, wearing a hospital gown. He is covered with two white blankets. He is hollering his head off. . . . A cleaning lady vacuums around him.*
> Observation: *Down the hallway the new patient . . . sits in her wheelchair. She is tied, with a sheet, to the handrail. She reaches for and pleads with everyone who passes by (to untie her).*

This newly admitted patient spent most of her first few days pleading with staff to untie her. As time passed, however, her objections waned. Below is a later observation of the same female patient.

> Observation: *A little further down the hallway an aide struggles to tie a sheet, which is wrapped around the waist of [a] . . . wheelchair patient (Ms. Ruth), to the hallway handrail. The patient is not cooperating.*
> MRS. RUTH: No! No! I want to go this way! (points down the hall)
> Observation: *There is no response from the aide.*
> MRS. RUTH: No! Let's go this way. (points) Please! (points) No! (pause) Let's get it going.
> Observation: *There is no response from the aide. She finishes tying the sheet and goes into the medication room. The patient struggles to move her wheelchair from the handrail for a few moments. Then she gives up and sits quietly.*

Some long-term patients offered no resistance at all. It is unclear to what degree this lack of response was related to prior unsuccessful attempts at resistance.

> Observation: *In the lounge I see two unidentified aides restraining Ms. Lyndon in her wheelchair. They twist and then wrap a sheet around her, tying it from behind. At first, she simply looks bewildered. Then, after the sheet is tied, she drops her head into her hands. They finish and leave. She remains there, motionless.*

Others, although restrained regularly, still struggled to free themselves.

> Note: *Television lounge.*
> MR. MCLAUGHLIN: Oh, open this thing up somebody!
> Observation: *Mr. McLaughlin wants out of his wheelchair. He has spent several minutes trying to get the posey off. He goes on to yell words I can't make any sense of.*
> MS. DONNER: Oh, you get it even if you don't want it.[5]

As the comment above by Ms. Donner indicates, some patients, even those cognitively impaired, regarded restraints as invasive. Most were not able to free themselves; the example below is an exception.

> Observation: *[An upper staff member] contributes with the description of an encounter she had earlier today. A patient was brought down*

from the sixth floor. It was a male patient, restrained in a geri-chair. She went to take the desk off the front. He said, "No, I can do that." Then he proceeded to unhook the desk. [The upper staff member] said, "You know how to do that?" The patient answered, "That's the first thing you learn to do when you come in a place like this."

More typically, patients' attempts to free themselves from restraints failed; at times such attempts put them in uncomfortable, and even hazardous, situations.[6]

Observation: *[Mr. McLaughlin] is tied in his wheelchair with a vest posey. He has the right shoulder strap worked part way down his right arm. Because of that, the posey is pulled tightly across his Adam's apple.*
Note: *Conversation with Nurse Biggs and Ms. Baker (an aide) in the staff lounge.*
NURSE BIGGS: Mr. Anderson tried to hang himself. (sarcastically)
OBSERVER: Hang himself?
NURSE BIGGS: Yeah. He can get himself out of bed, but he can't get himself out of the posey. So he gets his whole body out of bed and he hangs there with that thing tied around his neck.

Cognitive impairment appeared to prevent many restrained patients from even understanding the means by which their movements were restricted.

Observation: *I turn around and head for Ms. Donner's room. She's sitting in her wheelchair with her shoes off, struggling to get out of her posey. . . . She thinks that she needs to get herself out of her dress in order to get out of the [wheel]chair.*

Most of these patients did not understand why they were being restrained. Whether this was ever explained to them is unclear, but we never heard any such explanations being given.

OBSERVER: I've heard you're not too happy being in the wheelchair.
MS. DONNER: No. Uh-uh.
OBSERVER: Why are you in the wheelchair? Do you know?
MS. DONNER: Yes. Uh. Huh? Yes, they tell me . . . Uh . . .
OBSERVER: I hear you got pretty angry last night because they put you to bed and then put the bars up. You couldn't get out?

Ms. Donner: I was.
Observer: You were mad?
Ms. Donner: Uh-huh.
Observer: Why did they put the bars up? Do you know?
Ms. Donner: Uh-uh. No.

Whatever they understood about the reasons for and mechanics of the various restraints, even the most impaired individuals appeared to dislike immobilization. Sometimes they framed this quite dramatically.

> Observation: *[An upper staff member] refers to a patient [who] was quite confused. He used to sit, restrained in his geri-chair, and talk on an imaginary telephone. He would say things like, "Help! Is this the police? You've got to come and rescue me. They are holding me prisoner here."*

Impaired patients, unable to understand the reasons for their restraint and unable to free themselves, sometimes responded aggressively to staff attempts to restrain them.

> Observation: *Ms. Linley (a nurse) tells a story about Ms. Donner, who hit Ms. Laughren (an aide) in the arm this morning when Ms. Laughren tried to put the posey on.*

Staff occasionally worked together when restraining patients who were likely to resist.

> Observation: *Nurse Taylor and Ms. Baker (an aide) put Ms. Donner into a geri-chair. She resisted. Ms. Baker stood behind the geri-chair and held the patient's arms straight up into the air while Nurse Taylor fastened the desk onto the front of the chair.*

Line staff, in general, tended to support the use of restraints, particularly with problem patients.

Observer: I saw Mr. Viancia roll himself down the hallway. That's the first time I've seen him do that.
Ms. Marshall (an aide): Fortunately, he's usually in a geri-chair.

However, occasionally, even the line staff felt that restraints were used unnecessarily.

> NURSE SMITH: Now, if you just take your time and speak slowly, you can get Ms. Donner to do anything. It's just a matter of knowing how to handle her.

Upper staff, generally, did not view restraints (either geri-chairs or posies) as positively as line staff.

> OBSERVER: What determines whether a patient is put into a geri-chair or a wheelchair?
> US–02: Whether you want them to follow you around or not.
> OBSERVER: If you don't want them mobile you give them a geri-chair?
> US–02: Yes, because they're harder to push. A person can't move a geri-chair by themselves.

Indeed, some upper staff saw them as harmful.

> US–02: It's tough to break that mold that whenever you are told that someone falls a lot at home. . . . It seems to be a mindset so that when they get here, and we don't want them to fall anymore, it's restraints or chairs. . . . One of my big goals is to change that somehow, so that we do not confine as many people to wheelchairs as we do. . . . Not only with the patients, but with the families who are afraid that they (patients) will fall again. And with the whole staff and their fear of lawsuits. You know the legal profession has really tricked us into believing that restraints are really the answer to preventing problems, while all they really do is bring them on more.

In discussing Ms. Donner, who was walking when we started our observations but was restrained late in the observation period, the same upper staff member described the restraint as promoting her deterioration.

> US–02: I knew her (Ms. Donner) probably about four years ago. Then she was in here again six months ago. This lady was sharp. . . . She started out in the residential area, and then she came up here. In just the short time that she's been in this chair, she's gotten problems in her knees. She can't stand fully erect anymore. She has a little bit of a bend. . . . I don't know if they (line staff) felt that she was unsafe to walk by herself since she was dependent, and this was their answer to safety. "Let's put her in a chair." . . . I suppose that they don't want her standing by herself, and the answer to that is restraint.
> OBSERVER: Does she still have to be taken to the bathroom each time?

> US: Yes, that's correct. Hopefully she will still remember and be mentally aware when she needs to go to the bathroom.
> OBSERVER: Do you think her being in a chair will promote incontinence?
> US: That's exactly what I'm saying. I think that this chair business and the restraint business is a way of bringing on incontinence. It's a tough issue because there are no easy answers. You would like to not have to come up with this package answer since each resident and patient is different. You should cater to what their mental status is and what you think is appropriate for them. . . . And it's real tough to get staff to do that, especially when the budget is real low.

Occasionally the conflicting views were openly discussed.

> Observation: *She [nurse] goes into room 3012 and closes the door behind her. An aide follows her, carrying a hospital gown. Nurse Hastings and Upper Staff–02 continue to talk.*
> MS. HASTINGS: Does she [new patient] get a posey?
> US–02: Yes, a vest posey . . . another posey. (sounds disgusted)
> MS. HASTINGS: Look . . . anything that makes my work easier is fine with me.

Sometimes these disagreements led to conflicting procedures for managing patients.

> US–03: Every time she (Ms. Baker) came back from physical therapy they wouldn't put her back to bed and she was so tired. . . . So they (patients) sit there and all they can do is drop their heads down and fall asleep. . . . They are totally dependent on someone else. [When I] let her lay down in bed, I got criticized for doing it. "US, you know she just got up," or "She just came back from [physical therapy]." I said, "I understand that, but the woman is tired." Pt–40 did not want her side bars up. I took the plunge and tried it with them down. But the staff was not willing to do that. I'd go back in an hour later and find them up.

This conflict was not fundamentally about liability nor did it reflect the moral superiority of one group over another. Despite Nurse Hastings' comments above, both groups were worried about the patient's well-being and, based on their perspective, convinced that using or limiting the use of restraints was best for patients. The line staff were responsible for the enforcement of the routine restrictions and the maintenance of order. They thought, given their daily routine and staff limitations, that the only way to maintain order and protect patients' health was to use restraints. The upper staff, on the other hand, tended to view restraints primarily as a medical and psychological matter. They could see a variety of good reasons to refrain from using restraints and did not consider the line staff's difficulty with maintaining order and rules as a legitimate reason. They tended to believe that if the line staff were more willing to talk with patients they could usually avoid the use of restraints.

Many families supported the use of restraints; some specifically required their use.

> US–03: When he (Mr. Corzin) came the daughter informed us of what he was like at Woodhaven. And she wanted us to put side bars up. I mean we had specific instructions from that family.
> Observation: *On the wall is taped a note. It reads, "This is Ms. Woodland's daughter requesting that she be in a geri-chair all the time. No wheelchair, please."*

Others, while not desiring their use, seemed to sympathize with one argument that staff had made for their use.

> FAMILY: Going back two or three years, they (nursing home staff) were concerned that he (uncle) would fall and hurt himself. So they preferred to keep him confined. . . . I can understand the concerns of the staff. No matter what I say, somebody else is gonna sue them. If you wanna talk about the social impact of litigation. . . . It's a shame that he's not the only one that was held down for fear of hurting himself. Society tries to have this perfect environment where nobody gets hurt. Yet real life is not that way. . . . In the years we have been dealing with nursing homes, I see that as a problem. The home—to protect itself—has to become unduly restrictive with respect to the patients' desire to ambulate.

Conclusion

Line staff used physical redirection and restraints to contend with a variety of problems. In most instances, line staff used restraints and physical redirection because they felt they were necessary to protect patients from falls and other injuries. However, in some cases upper staff disagreed about the appropriateness of these measures. This may, in part, reflect greater training on the part of upper staff and therefore a greater awareness of the limited effectiveness of restraints. However, it seems that a substantial part of the disagreement arose from the line staff's concern with the maintenance of order, efficient task completion, and the enforcement of rules.

What is clear is that the consistent use of force is both caused by and a cause of the staff's inability to get patients to cooperate with many tasks. In order to gain control of the situation the staff felt they needed to use force. The staff's difficulty in convincing patients to follow their requests was exacerbated by the patients' cognitive impairments. This was reflected in the fact that almost every instance of physical redirection or restraint occurred with severely cognitively impaired patients.

Whether the differential use and acceptance of physical redirection and restraint can be changed through training in other techniques of patient management is unclear. An alternative possibility is to reduce the types of restrictions that line staff must maintain and lower the expectations about the preservation of physical safety. These issues cannot be resolved with the research methods used in this study.

NOTES

1. Force can be used in more or less justifiable forms. This will depend on factors such as whether the participants have agreed to the use of force, whether the user is exercising force for which she holds societally authorized authority, whether the use of force violates other values such as dignity, and whether the institution's goals are societally legitimated.

2. It should be noted that this description is of only the intermediate and skilled units. We did not observe either physical redirection or restraints in the residential area.

3. It is an open question whether the use of behavioral methods, rather than force, would be a more ethically justifiable method for controlling patients' behavior.

4. We have argued throughout this report that this view is mistaken. Restraints were, by and large, only used in severely cognitively impaired patients who had little capability to act autonomously. Still, restraints did seem to preclude whatever minimal capacity for autonomous behavior the patient might have had. Moreover, there are other reasons for being concerned about the use of restraints—for example, their effect on patient safety or dignity.

5. One needs to be careful how one interprets the statements of cognitively impaired patients. It is often quite difficult to impute cognitive states to them on the basis of their behavior as their behavior so often seems totally random.

6. In fact, many medical experts now argue that physical restraints put patients at an increased, rather than a decreased risk of physical harm (Evans, Strumpf 1989).

11

Summary and Implications for Long-Term Care

Throughout the last seven chapters, we have sought to describe the various ways in which the institutional structures of a nursing facility affect elderly residents' autonomy. One way of summarizing these very diverse findings is to consider the applicability of Erving Goffman's notion of "total institution" to nursing homes and its ramifications for autonomy. We will then analyze the appropriateness of autonomy for guiding health care professionals' care of nursing home residents and argue that a more basic, related value, such as dignity or respect for humans, has greater relevance for the care of the severely demented. Finally, drawing in part on our observations in the residential care setting, we will suggest some ways in which nursing homes can be modified in order to promote the ability of patients and residents to live autonomously in long-term care settings.

Life on the Nursing Side—A "Total Institution"?

Our central argument in this study is that one's ability to direct one's own life is profoundly and directly affected by the social context in which one exists. People live within institutions which, to varying degrees, structure their values, choices, and world view. In his landmark study, *Asylums*, Goffman takes a similar position regarding the influence of societal institutions on individuals' behavior (Goffman 1961). Moreover, he describes a group of social structures, called "total institutions," that exert a particularly pernicious effect on autonomy:

> Total institutions disrupt or defile precisely those actions that in civil society have the role of attesting to the actor and those in his presence that he has some command over his world—that he is a person with "adult" self-determination, autonomy and freedom of action (Goffman 1961:43).

Among the different types of organizations Goffman classifies as "total institutions" are mental hospitals, nunneries, military training camps, boys' preparatory schools, concentration camps, orphanages, and "old age homes." What each of these seemingly diverse institutions has in common is the way in which they affect individuals' lives.

> A basic social arrangement in modern society is that the individual tends to sleep, play, and work in different places with different co-participants, under different authorities, and without an over-all rational plan. The central features of total institutions can be described as a breakdown of the barriers ordinarily separating these three spheres of life (Goffman 1961:5–6).

We believe that the nursing home that we studied approximates Goffman's conception of a "total institution" in many ways.[1] While nursing homes do not meet every characteristic of a total institution, they exemplify enough attributes to be classified as a total institution. As Goffman himself notes, in defining total institutions,

> None of the elements I will describe seems peculiar to total institutions, and none seems to be shared by every one of them; what is distinctive about total institutions is that each exhibits to an intense degree many items in this family of attributes (Goffman 1961: 5).

Reviewing Goffman's writings on the subject, we have identified 15 observable features of total institutions. Reviewing our findings in terms of these characteristics will be helpful in explicating the effect of nursing homes on elderly participants' ability to live autonomously.

1. *Entry rituals, including stripping of an individual's private identity and categorizing and processing an individual's life, such as history taking, fingerprinting, etc, are common.* Once a person was admitted to the nursing home, she went from being an unique individual with a long and complex psychosocial history to being a patient who was largely known by her medical history. Moreover, patients were not able to bring their furniture or most of their possessions to the nursing home. Their rooms were furnished almost identically, further stripping individuals of their private identity. The major exception to the recategorizing of individuals as patients was that, if they were able to assist in dressing themselves, they were

allowed to wear their own clothes. However, most patients lived in hospital gowns, nightgowns, and robes.

2. *Locational dedifferentiation: All aspects of life are conducted in the same place.* Patients in the intermediate and skilled care units rarely left the nursing home. Patients ate, slept, and spent their waking hours all within the same building. The more mentally impaired an individual was, the more limiting the space in which the individual lived. Patients could spend days on end going between their rooms, the bathroom, and either the TV lounges or dining room for meals.

3. *Dedifferentiation of authority: In "total institutions" there is a single, unspecialized authority hierarchy.* For most purposes, there were only two groups in the nursing home—patients and staff. Staff, whether nurses, aides, or therapists, were seen as having final authority to make all decisions in the nursing home. Thus staff-patient interactions consisted almost exclusively of patients asking staff for permission and never the reverse. Whenever there was disagreement between patients and staff about what should be done, staff's viewpoint dominated.

4. *Each phase of the patients' daily activity is carried on in the immediate company of a large group of others, all of whom are treated alike.* Unlike persons outside the nursing home, patients did not choose the people with whom to spend their days. Except for family visits, patients spent their entire day in the company of other patients and staff with whom they had no prior personal ties and who were selected by others. Organizational procedures rather than individual patient wants and needs guided staff behavior. Thus, cognitively intact patients were not preferentially roomed with other intact patients, and no attention was paid to who wanted to room with whom. Staff treatment of patients seemed based more on the task at hand than the individual characteristics of the patients. While there was some differentiation between staff's responses based on patients' cognitive status, the major determinant of their response to patients' requests was whether the requests interfered with staff routines. Staff restrictions also focused primarily on safeguarding patient health (defined in general, rather than individual terms) and institutional efficiency rather than individual patient requests or needs.

5. *Daily activities are tightly scheduled by staff with little individual variation permitted.* Patients' daily routines—their arising in the morning, their mealtimes, and their bedtimes—were highly scheduled by staff. Staff structured the entire day of cognitively impaired patients: their recreational activities, their daily routines, even when they could go to the bathroom. Even cognitively intact patients had no say in when they got up or the order in which their morning activities occurred. Although less structure was

imposed on the rest of cognitively aware patients' time, we still found little patient-directed activity, perhaps reflecting the setting's influence on patients' ability to autonomously organize their lives.

6. *Violations of privacy are common.* As noted in Chapter 8, there was minimal privacy in the nursing home. Rooms were shared, doors were open, and almost anyone could obtain unrestricted access to patients' space. We also found that patients' privacy of information, of possessions, and of body were routinely violated in the nursing home. This was true for both competent and incompetent patients.

7. *There is a small group of staff members whose primary role is to ensure enforcement of the rules.* Line staff did not so much enforce rules as maintain a routine. Without the rebellious inmates that one might find in a prison, a mental hospital, or even an orphanage, staff's primary role became physically assuring compliance with the organizational routine.

8. *Severe restrictions on patient contact with the outside world, particularly at entry.* There were no formal restrictions on communication with the outside world. Such communication was, however, difficult in practice. Most patients did not have or could not afford a personal telephone, and the only public telephones were in the staff lounges, which required staff permission for use. The most extensive communication with the outside world was likely to occur shortly after entry, when contacts with the community were most intact. However, the absence of restrictions made little real difference. Most patients were incapable of extensive communication with the outside world.[2] Moreover, as time passed, patients had greater difficulty maintaining significant relationships with people outside of the nursing home. Leaving the facility for any reason was, therefore, an uncommon event that acquired a special significance.[3]

9. *Line staff function to control patient communication to higher staff.* Communication with the patients' physicians was mediated almost entirely through the line nursing staff. Physicians visited rarely, and typically changed medication and other medical orders at the staff's request. However, no effort was made to interfere with patient communication to the people we have called "upper staff." Again, however, it is important to remember that many of the patients were cognitively unable to sustain complex conversations with either the upper or line staff.[4]

10. *Patients and staff view each other through narrow hostile stereotypes.* We have already noted that line staff tend to view patients in hostile ways. In general, staff viewed patients as demented, unrealistic, and demanding. Patients also tended to view all staff as alike and made few distinctions among them. Both sides frequently spoke of the other as *they.* That said, there was considerable fondness for some of the patients, particularly

among the upper staff who did not have to manage the day-to-day details of body care.

11. *Patients were excluded from making plans about themselves.* Even cognitively intact patients were not invited to care conference or discharge planning meetings. We saw no evidence that patients were included in such planning in any manner except that they were informed when discharges or transfers were planned.

12. *Rituals characterized by patient deference toward staff develop in total institutions.* We did not see any rituals in which patients showed their deference to the staff.

13. *Patients must request staff permission for routine activities and tools.* Patients' physical disability required that they routinely ask for staff assistance in accomplishing most tasks. Still, staff control over the facilities extended beyond this biological necessity. For example, staff permission was required to use the telephone since the only functioning outside telephone was in the staff lounge. As noted previously, patient interaction with staff consisted almost entirely of requests.

14. *Discrediting reports about patients commonly spread through staff ranks.* We saw many instances of this activity. Staff spread damaging information to each other and to our observers. Often this information was not based on direct observation but was hearsay obtained from other staff. To a significant degree the medical records served as a repository for this sort of information.

15. *All activities are brought together into a single rational plan designed to fulfill the official aims of the institution.* This, of course, is true of almost any formal organization but not of informal groups. This formal organization had a rational plan organized around the value of health. In nursing homes, because of the chronicity of illnesses, this translates into an emphasis on basic bodily functions and activities of daily living such as eating, bathing, and toileting. Consistent with this emphasis on bodily health, the normative expectations of patient and staff were defined by the traditional doctor-patient relationship. Staff were, on the basis of their medical expertise, seen as the decision-makers. It was their job to define what was good for the patient and to structure the patient's care.[5] Elderly individuals living in the nursing home were seen as "sick" patients. Their job was, therefore, to comply with the staff's orders in an attempt to "get better."

The Impact of Nursing Homes on Autonomy

Whatever the positive attributes of a total institution dedicated to promoting bodily well-being, it is detrimental to patient autonomy. This is true regardless of the conception of autonomy that one holds, although as we will argue, its impact on autonomy as "consistency" is the most critical for understanding nursing home residents' lives.

Free Action

The "institutionalization" of nursing home patients severely limited their ability to take free action. The highly structured aspects of patients' lives limited their ability to choose what they wanted to do. For example, patients had no choices about such basic matters as when they were to get up, when they were to eat, and when they were to go to sleep. Moreover, because of their physical limitations, staff help was often necessary for patients to carry out their free choices. Staff, however, were not predisposed to helping patients do this, particularly if it required substantial staff effort or interfered with the staff routines.

Still, cognitively intact patients were able to make a fair number of decisions and, in general, the staff respected these autonomous free actions. The problem for these patients was that most of these decisions dealt with fairly minor issues such as what to eat for a meal.

> Observation: *Then an aide comes to the table and picks up Ms. Gartner and Ms. Castra's dietary cards. Ms. Gartner speaks to her.*
> Ms. Gartner: Hey let me have meat sauce instead of that other stuff.
> Ms. Hartman (the aide): OK. Instead of meatballs?
> Ms. Gartner: Yeah.
> Observation: *Ms. Hartman takes the pen out of her pocket and makes a change on the dietary card.*

While the nursing home respected cognitively intact patients' free action, the limited number of meaningful options decreased the value of their actions. By restricting the range and number of options that patients can choose between, the nursing home environment renders patients' autonomous choices increasingly irrelevant.

Staff response to cognitively impaired patients' attempts to act autonomously was markedly different. Their requests were usually ignored and almost never honored; their actions were often challenged by the staff. This behavior is understandable, if not justified, because the severe cognitive deficits of some patients raises the question of whether their actions were truly intentional or not. What is more disturbing is that staff did not expend much energy trying to determine if patients' actions were intentional. Staff seemed to assume that if a patient was impaired that all of her actions were not autonomous and therefore not worthy of respect. This assumption seems unwarranted. A moderately impaired patient may be unable to autonomously make complicated decisions or act in a consistent manner over time to realize long-term goals, but still be capable of deciding what she wants to eat, or when she wants to go to bed. Thus, viewed from the perspective of autonomy as free action, many moderately to severely demented patients have at least some capacity for autonomous activity.[6] Unfortunately, staff were unable or unwilling, given the institutional demands placed upon them, to make these distinctions.

Effective Deliberation

It is difficult to assess the effect of the nursing home environment on autonomy as effective deliberation. At the onset of this study we somewhat naively expected to observe many major decisions of the kind that are commonly discussed in the ethics literature. Unfortunately, such decisions were rare in nursing home patients' lives. For example, during our observation we did not see one patient or family confronted with a decision regarding life-sustaining treatment. Patients' lives consisted of many small decisions rather than the type of discrete decisions with major benefits and harms assumed by autonomy as effective deliberation.

The only decisions that at all approximated the type assumed by this model of autonomy concerned issues of discharge and post-discharge planning. However, even these decisions were relatively uncommon. An analysis of autonomy that focuses on effective deliberation will, therefore, not be very helpful in understanding the impact of nursing homes on the elderly's ability to live autonomously.[7]

When these decisions occurred, we found little evidence that the staff encouraged patient input, much less effective deliberation. In many cases, decisions related to major treatments or placement were made in weekly discharge and planning meetings. These meetings were attended by most of the upper staff but not patients, families, or line staff. Consequently patients were given no opportunity to learn about the decision-making process. The other place where major treatment or placement decisions were made was the weekly care conferences held on each unit. Here again, patients, regardless of their cognitive abilities, were not invited to participate. Thus, we saw no effort to respect or to promote patients' ability to effectively deliberate and make autonomous decisions.[8]

Consistency

The most useful conception of autonomy in the nursing home setting is concerned with the structure of patients' lives rather than discrete decisions. A conception of autonomy that deals with the patterns and structure of a patient's life is more relevant to the real experience of patients in long-term care. If an autonomous agent is thought of as someone who has a strong sense of identity, someone whose activities are consistent with her personal history, who has a coherent self-directed set of commitments and involvements in daily life, and who has a sense of directedness toward future goals, it is possible to see how the structure of nursing home care affects patients' autonomy in meaningful ways. Unfortunately, it is here that nursing homes had the most pernicious effect on patient autonomy. The "total institutional" characteristics of the nursing home acted to inhibit patients' interest in developing any goals or interest that could, in any sense of the word, be described as theirs.

When individuals are admitted to nursing homes they lose their identity as independent agents and become "patients." What makes nursing homes so problematic from the point of view of autonomy is their tendency to make elderly individuals stop living their own lives. We saw few individuals who expressed goals of any sort—short- or long-term. The institutionalization of patients' lives seems to have resulted in their losing interest in the things that made them unique individuals.

The nursing home staff did little to support patients' autonomy. Line staff saw their job as primarily ensuring that patients' bodily needs were cared for. More importantly, the medical model of the doctor-patient relationship, which defines role relations in the nursing home, specifies a patient role that undercuts personal individuality. In this model, health care providers are supposed to tell patients what to do, not help them develop their own interests. Patients are expected to follow health care providers' direction, not act independently. Helping patients retain their autonomy is just not part of the medical model.

Combined with a disregard for allowing patients to make decisions was a substantial limiting of patient liberties. Staff paid little attention to whom the patients had been, much less to allowing them the space and options to develop new interests and goals. The few areas in which the patients were allowed to make decisions were peripheral to their self-development. Patients' ability to develop interests and goals, their ability individuate themselves, was thus severely hampered.

Autonomy and Demented Patients

An important caveat should be added to our conclusion that the nursing home environment is not conducive to patient autonomy. Unfortunately, for many patients autonomy was an irrelevant value. A significant number of patients did not have the capacity for autonomous activity, regardless of the conception of autonomy used. While we did not, and perhaps could not, definitively measure what proportion of the patients were capable of autonomous action, staff judged the large majority of patients to be incapable of rational decision-making.

Since any conception of autonomy requires a minimum level of cognitive functioning, efforts to promote or respect the autonomy of some of these patients makes little sense. One must have, at the very least, a conception of oneself as an agent who can affect the external world through one's action. One must, in other words, have some conscious control over one's behavior. Many patients were so demented that it was unclear whether there was any connection between their behavior and their "self." One moment a patient would want something to eat, the next she would want nothing to eat, the next she would be ranting incoherently.

More complicated conceptions of autonomy require even more cognitive functioning. Autonomy as effective deliberation requires that the individual have the cognitive ability to understand the situation at hand, to assess risks and benefits, and to make a decision. Autonomy as "consistency" requires the capacity to maintain enduring goals and desires that persist over time. Many patients exhibited none of these cognitive skills. These patients' days were spent largely lying in bed or sitting in a wheelchair, often mumbling unintelligibly. Their speech and activity showed no sign of either conscious, goal-directed behavior or the ability to weigh risks and benefits rationally.[9]

Attempts to promote these patients' autonomy would be a serious mistake for several reasons. First, to a certain extent, to be autonomous means to be responsible for one's choices. However, these patients are unable to control their behavior in any significant way. To hold them responsible or punish them for their behavior seems unfair. One should no more hold a severely demented patient responsible for her unintelligible desires than one would punish a six-month-old for urinating in her diaper. Second, according to most ethical theories, one has a prima facie duty not to interfere with another's autonomous behavior. Thus, we often allow individuals to make what we might consider bad choices out of a respect for autonomy. The severely demented, however, do not have the ability to develop a life plan, or to assess what is in their best interest. Respecting their behavior as autonomous requires that we respect a value they do not and cannot have. Moreover, this respect may result in the demented patient seriously harming himself—for example, the demented patient who attempts to climb over his bed rails without help and falls and breaks a bone.

Autonomy, therefore, should have little role in determining health care professionals' duties toward the seriously demented. —We need to appeal to a different value to determine the responsibilities of those who care for patients whose cognitive capacities are severely diminished.

In traditional Judeo-Christian theology, respect for the dignity of human beings would serve this role. According to this theory, human beings were created in God's image. To treat an individual in an undignified manner was, therefore, a sin against God. This meant that all human beings, regardless of their ability to act autonomously, must be treated with dignity.[10]

In a world in which religion is increasingly divorced from everyday life, religious teachings no longer guarantee respect for the demented.[11] We need to develop a more secular basis for respecting the dignity of the human body. Ronald Dworkin believes that a right not to suffer indignity requires that all humans, regardless of their mental or physical capacities, have a right not to be treated in ways that, in the particular culture or community to which they belong, are seen as showing disrespect (Dworkin 1986).[12]

This right to dignity requires that we remember that even demented patients remain persons (Dworkin 1986).[13] We mark their continued moral standing by insisting that nothing be done to them that, in our community's definition of respect, demeans their irrevocably human nature. This value should help explain our discomfort with some of the things that we reported the line staff did when caring for mentally incompetent patients, eg, using physical violence to ensure compliance and violating patient privacy.[14]

The OBRA Regulations: A Regulatory Solution?

Neither we nor many other writers about the current conditions in nursing homes have been very enthusiastic about the impact of federal and state regulations. After the completion of our field work, a new series of regulations, usually referred to as the OBRA regulations (after the Omnibus Budget Reconciliation Act of 1987 that mandated them), went into effect. While the regulations are complex and not easily summarized, some sections clearly reflect a concern with some of the issues which we have discussed in this volume. Two parts are directly relevant.

One section concerns the training of nurses' aides. Since aides are the staff members with the most contact with residents (as OBRA refers to people whom we, following the usage at the facility we studied, have referred to as "patients"), such training is directed at the right target. However, since the focus on the body is part of the problem, the content of the training is at best mixed. The regulations specify that training must be done in basic nursing skills; personal care skills; cognitive, behavioral, and social care; basic restorative services; and residents' rights. Unless training in residents' rights is imaginatively and persuasively done, there is a substantial chance that this sort of training will increase the focus on caring for the residents' bodies rather than supporting their independence.

The impact of the rules on autonomy depends largely on the sections on residents' rights. In some ways the new rights are directly on target. They include rights

1. to be free from restraints,
2. to privacy,
3. to participate in resident groups,
4. to voice grievances,
5. to participate in activities,
6. to be fully informed about changes in treatment and living situation.

Without suggesting that these are not important provisions, we must note that all of them have significant limits.

1. Freedom from restraints is qualified by the exception that they may be used to "ensure the physical safety of the resident or other residents." Since we rarely saw them used for any other purpose, this is a very limited right.
2. The right to privacy is vaguely worded and there is a specific exemption to say that it does not assure a private room.
3. The right to participate in resident groups would mean little to most of our patients unless such groups were organized and encouraged by some other source since few patients seemed eager to interact with others. Indeed, many of our patients would probably prefer the "right not to participate."
4. The right to voice grievances does not assure that they will be taken seriously.
5. The right to participate in activities was almost always supported by line staff who encouraged patients to do anything that took them off the floor.
6. The right to be informed of changes does not provide the corresponding right to have any influence on the decision.

Finally, it needs to be pointed out that none of the rights contain a significant exemption for people who are incompetent to participate. As should be apparent from previous chapters, any such rules that make no such exemptions must, of necessity, seem like unreasonable bureaucratic impingements to those who are supposed to implement them. Even the best intentioned efforts to implement such rules will soon break down into absurdity.

Applying the Lessons of Residential Area to the Nursing Home

How to increase patients' autonomy in the nursing home setting is a difficult medical, social, and economic problem. Our purpose is not to develop a detailed public policy for the care of elderly patients. We are not willing or able to propose a new set of OBRA rights. We wish only to point out the effect of current policies on the institutionalized elderly's lives, particularly their ability to act autonomously. Still, the following points seem clear.

1. Autonomy is only one of several values that guide behavior in the nursing home setting. We have noted how the staff's attempts to promote their conceptionalization of beneficence affected patients' lives. Efforts to maximize patients' bodily function often required limiting autonomy. Similarly, staff seemed to value institutional efficacy more than patient autonomy. Allowing patients' freedom to structure their own lives, it was felt, would require more intensive staffing patterns. Efforts to promote autonomy will require balancing competing values. Current policies, such as routine use of restraints, favor body care and institutional efficacy over promoting patients' autonomy. It may be that allowing patients increased autonomy will result in patients' safety being at higher risk or in a decrease in institutional efficacy. When developing public policy, we must remain aware of these trade-offs and face them in an explicit manner. We may determine that these trade-offs are worthwhile in cognitively intact patients but not in the severely demented patients in whom it is impossible to promote autonomy in a significant way.

2. We need to separate the medical care function from the residential function of nursing homes. Those staff whose job it is to facilitate patients' day-to-day living do not need nursing training. Those staff whose job it is to provide nursing care do not need to have daily responsibility for most patients beyond implementing treatment. Nursing care, like medical care and social services, can be a specialized, as-needed, function. Most important, we need to abolish the idea that elderly people who are in some way disabled are full-time patients and should "follow (caregivers) orders" full-time. Current efforts to conceptualize long-term care as a branch of the hospitality industry rather than as medical care seems like a good start in

this direction.[15] This different conception of staff and resident roles seems to explain many of the differences between nursing home care and the care of the residents. In the independent living setting, sustaining autonomous functioning, not health care, seemed the dominant value among line staff. Rather than viewing themselves as medical personnel, monitors saw their role as helping the residents live their lives as the residents defined them. Of course, there were significant differences in the average levels of mobility and cognitive capacities of the elderly in the two settings, but there was also a fair degree of overlap. The clearest difference between the two settings was that the nursing home was organized around a medical model, while the residential setting was seen as providing a place where residents could live autonomously.

3. We need to do a better job of separating patients according to cognitive ability. The needs of very demented patients are quite different from the needs of those whose physical impairments limit their ability to live without substantial help. Any staff, no matter how well trained and thoughtful, will need to rely on routines and will, to some extent, try to treat all cases similarly. Thus, it seems counterproductive to mix together elderly individuals whose care should require radically different orientations.

4. Numerous times over the past decade commentators have noted that nursing home regulation regulates the wrong things. Administrators who must spend all of their time managing the completeness of nursing records cannot focus on making the lives of their charges fuller and more independent. Nursing home regulations, as we saw in Chapter 2, grew out of the desire to upgrade care. However, this upgrading was based on the hospital model of care and is thus focused on maintaining sanitation and safety rather than personal independence. Whatever their other virtues, from the point of view of promoting autonomy, current regulations are part of the problem, not part of the solution.

5. Beyond these general suggestions there are many more specific ways in which nursing homes can be modified in order to promote their residents' autonomy. These include major reductions in the use of restraints, improved privacy, flexibility of scheduling, and substantial modifications of line staff's training and job descriptions.

In short, we want to suggest that promoting the autonomy of the elderly in long-term care requires a minor revolution rather than just tinkering at the margins of current practice. Such a change will be difficult. It requires major modifications in the financing, regulation, administration and staffing of long-term care for the elderly. But if we take seriously the humanity of our elderly citizens who need this sort of care, we can do no less.

NOTES

1. Shield (1988:98) suggests that there are important limitations to the application of this model to the nursing home. In general her critique seems correct, but most of it is not directly pertinent to our purposes here.

2. Of course we did not see most of these patients until long after they were admitted, and we don't know how much of their cognitive incompetence was related to their isolation from the outside world.

3. See Gubrium (1975) for an excellent description of the ritual character of leaving the facility for a brief visit.

4. Another relevant factor is that, unlike most total institutions, line staff contained some full professional nurses whom the "upper staff" felt that they could not simply order around.

5. It is important to note that upper staff did not seem to hold significantly different values. The administrative staff and the non-line professionals expressed considerable concern about patient autonomy. Unfortunately, upper staff were not as important as lower staff in defining patients' daily lives, and line staff were not concerned with autonomy.

6. Moderately impaired patients' ability to effectively deliberate should also be thought of as a decision-specific rather than as a global attribute. Unfortunately, we have no data concerning how staff thought about this aspect of autonomy.

7. Since most patients' cognitive abilities were very limited it is doubtful whether the institution could have helped patients effectively deliberate.

8. For incompetent patients, one might argue that involving the family in decisions would count as a proxy for patient involvement. In fact, families were involved in the weekly care conferences and upper staff did encourage them to state their preferences. However, for families to truly serve as proxy decision-makers they should, according to the ethics literature, reflect to caregivers what the patient would have wanted in the situations (Buchanan, Brock 1989). We saw no examples in which staff asked families to reflect the patient's preferences or where the family commented on what they thought the patient would want.

9. Of course it is possible that some of this is a response to the nursing home environment and that with a more stimulating environment they would do better. Presumably judgments about ability to function autonomously should be made at entry in a "generous" manner and changed only if it becomes apparent that the judgement was too optimistic.

10. The literature in this area is so wide and diverse as to be impossible to summarize. See, for example Troeltsch (1958).

11. The principle bioethicists commonly appeal to in guiding behavior for an incompetent patient is "substituted judgment." This principle states that one should do what the person would want us to do if she were currently competent. We are unsure how helpful this principle will be in guiding the day-to-day life of the severely demented nursing home patient. For example, would it require that because you used to love Beethoven, that we ought to take you, now severely demented, and force you to listen to Beethoven even if you told us to turn it off? A plausible interpretation would be that the principle is directing us to respect the patient's prior wishes about what she would want done if she should ever become severely demented. Unfortunately few persons have considered this in enough detail to be useful.

12. This right can be grounded in secular terms in one of two ways. First, one might argue that "a person's right to be treated with dignity . . . is the right that

others acknowledge that he has genuine evaluative interests, that is, that they acknowledge that he is the kind of creature, and has the moral standing, such that it is intrinsically important whether his life is a good one or bad one" (Dworkin 1986). Thus, even though one is cognitively impaired, what happens to him is important because it will affect the value or success of his life as a whole. The other argument for this value is not based on the impact that its violation will have on the severely demented. Instead this argument is based on the effect of the violation on the caregiver. Treating humans in this way reflects the kind of society we are. Moreover, this behavior may well affect our behavior towards less demented individuals. For a version of this argument see May (1985) and Kass (1985). For a critique of this view see Feinberg (1985).

13. We therefore, like Dworkin, deny that indignity is wrong because it is contrary to our experiential interests. As Dworkin points out, "The experiential theory of indignity, however, is unpersuasive, because it cannot explain central features of the use we make of the idea of indignity. Most of us think that slaves live in the ultimate indignity even if—particularly if—their subjugation is so complete that they believe their slavery appropriate and do not resent or otherwise suffer any special distress from it" (Dworkin 1986:59).

14. The exact definition of what it means to treat patients with dignity may be difficult to determine and is certainly beyond the scope of our task here. For our purposes it is enough to suggest the contours of such a right and to point out that this right was sometimes violated by line staff's care of the mentally impaired.

15. For example, see Wolfe (1989), which discusses several such recent attempts.

References

Abdellah FC (1978). The future of long-term care. *Bull NY Acad Med.*, 54(March): 24–41.

Agich GJ (1988). Autonomy and long term care. A study prepared for *The Retirement Research Foundation*.

Anderson NN, Stone LB (1969). Nursing homes: Research and public policy. *Gerontologist*. 9 (Autumn):214–223.

Appelbaum PS, Lidz CW, Meisel A (1987). *Informed Consent: Legal Theory and Clinical Practice*. New York: Oxford University Press.

Beauchamp TL, Childress JF (1989). *Principles of Biomedical Ethics*. New York: Oxford University Press.

Buchanan A, Brock B. (1989). *Deciding for Others*. Cambridge: Cambridge University Press.

Burt RA (1979). *Taking Care of Strangers*. New York: Free Press.

Callahan D (1984). Autonomy: A moral good, not a moral obsession. *Hastings Center Report*, 14:40–42.

Cassel CK, Hofland BF. (1988). Patient autonomy in long-term care: Is it possible? What does it mean? (unpublished manuscript).

Cassell EJ (1989). Autonomy and ethics in action. *NEngl Med.* 297(6):333–334.

Childress JF (1982). *Who Should Decide? Paternalism in Health Care*. New York: Oxford University Press. 250 pp.

Christman, J (1987). Autonomy: A defense of the split-level self. *South J Phil.* 25(3):281–193.

Christman J (1988). Constructing the inner citadel: Recent work on the concept of autonomy. *Ethics*. 99:109–124.

Christman J, ed (1989). *The Inner Citadel: Essays on Individual Autonomy*. New York: Oxford University Press.

Cohen ES (1985). Autonomy and Paternalism: Two goals in conflict. *Law Med Health Care*. 13(4).

Cole TR (1987). Class, culture and coercion: A historical perspective on longterm care. *Generations*. (Summer): 9–15.

Collopy BJ (1986). The Conceptually Problematic Status of Autonomy. A Study Prepared for The Retirement Research Foundation.

Collopy BJ (1988). Autonomy in long term care: Some crucial distinctions. *Gerontologist*. 28:10–17.

Duggan T, Gert B (1967). Voluntary abilities. *Am Phil Q.*, 4(2):127–135.

Durkheim, E (1951); Spaulding JA, Simpson G, trans. *Suicide*. Glencoe, IL: Free Press.

Dworkin G (1976). Autonomy and behavior control. *Hastings Center Report*, 6:23–28.

Dworkin G (1988). *The Theory and Practice of Autonomy*. Cambridge, U.K.: Cambridge University Press.

Dworkin R (1986). Philosophical issues in senile dementia. *A Report for the Office of Technology Assessment.*

Edwards RB (1988). Confidentiality and the professions. In: Edwards RB, Graber GC, Graber eds. *Bioethics*. San Diego: Harcourt Brace Jovanovich:72–81.

Englehart TH (1978). Moral autonomy and the polis: Response to Gerald Dworkin and Gregory Vlastos. In: Englehart TH, Callahan D (eds.) *Morals, Science, and Sociality.* Hastings-on-Hudson: The Hastings Center.

Evans LK, Strumpf NE (1989). Tying down the elderly: A review of the literature on physical restraint, *JAGS*, 37:65–74.

Faden, RR, Beauchamp TL (1986). *A History and Theory of Informed Consent.* New York: Oxford University Press.

Feinberg J (1985). *Offense to Others.* New York: Oxford University Press.

Feinberg J (1986). *Harm to Self.* Volume 3 of *The Moral Limits of Criminal Law.* New York: Oxford University Press.

Feinberg J (1989). Mistreatment of dead bodies. *Hasting Center Report*. 15:31–38.

Gartner A, Riessman F (1977). *Self-Help In The Human Services*. Jossey-Bass: San Francisco, CA.

Goffman E (1961). *Asylums: Essays on the social situation of mental patients and other inmates*. Garden City, N.J.: Anchor Books.

Gottlieb BH (1982). Mutual-help groups: Members' views of their benefits and of roles for professionals. In: Borman LD, Borck LE, Hess R, Pasquale FL, eds. *Helping People to Help Themselves: Self-Help and Prevention*. New York: Haworth Press.

Gubrium J (1975). *Living and Dying at Murray Manor.* New York: St Martin's Press. 99–104.

Hayworth L (1986). *Autonomy: An essay in philosophical psychology and ethics.* New Haven, CT: Yale University Press.

Hofland BF (1988). Autonomy in long term care: Background issues and a programmatic response. *Gerontologist*. 28:3–9.

Institute of Medicine, Committee on Nursing Home Regulation: *Improving the quality of care in nursing homes* (1986). Washington, DC: National Academy Press.

Kant I (1964); Paton HJ, trans. *Groundwork of the Metaphysic of Morals*. New York: Harper and Row.

Kahneman D, Tversky A (1982). Judgement under uncertainty: Heurestics and biases. In: Kahneman D, Slovic P, Tversky A., eds. *Judgment under uncertainty: Heuristics and biases*. Cambridge: Cambridge University Press, 2–23.

Kass LR (1985). *Toward a More Natural Science.* New York: The Free Press.
Katz J (1984). *The Silent World of Doctor and Patient.* New York: Free Press.
Komrad MS (1983). A Defence of medical paternalism: Maximizing patient autonomy. *J Med Ethics.* 9(1):38–44.
Landenson RF (1975). A theory of personal autonomy. *Ethics.* 86:30–48.
Lidz CW (1983). Informed consent in mental health treatment: A sociological perspective. *Behavioral Sciences and the Law.* 1:21–27.
Lidz CW, Meisel A, Zerubavel E, Carter M, Sestak R, Roth LH (1984). *Informed Consent: A Study of Psychiatric Decision-making.* New York: Guilford.
Lidz CW, Meisel A, Munetz M (1985). Chronic disease and patient participation. *Culture, Medicine and Psychiatry.* 9:1,1–17.
Lieberman MA (1979). Help seeking and self-help groups. In: Lieberman MA, Borman LD, eds. *Self-Help Groups For Coping with Crisis.* San Francisco CA: Jossey-Bass.
Lucas JL (1966). *Principles of Politics.* New York: Oxford University Press.
May W (1985). Attitudes toward the newly dead. *The Hastings Center Report* 1: 3–13.
McCullough L (1984). Medical care for elderly patients with diminished competence: An ethical analysis. *J Am Geri Soc.* 32:150–153.
Mendelson MA (1974). *Tender Loving Greed: How The Incredibly Lucrative Nursing Home "Industry" Is Exploiting America's Old People and Defrauding Us All.* New York: Alfred A. Knopf.
Merton R (1949). *Social Theory and Social Structure.* Glencoe IL: Free Press.
Mill JS (1955). *On Liberty.* Chicago: Henry Regnery.
Miller BL (1981). Autonomy and the refusal of lifesaving treatment. *Hasting Center Report.* 11(4):22–28.
Moody HR (1988). From informed consent to negotiated consent. *Gerontologist.* 28:64–70.
Mosca G (1939). *The Ruling Class.* New York: McGraw-Hill.
Nathanson v Kline, 186 Kan 393, 350. P2d 1093, 254 P2d 670 (1986).
Parsons T (1951). *The Social System.* Glencoe IL: Free Press. Chapter 10.
Parsons T (1958). Definitions of health and illness in the light of american values and social structure. In: Jaco EG, ed. *Patients, Physicians and Illness.* New York: The Free Press of Glencoe.
President's Commission for the Study of Ethical Problems in Medicine and Biomedical and Behavioral Research: *Making Health Care Decisions* (1982). Washington DC: US Government Printing Office.
Rauchlin, HS (1980). An analysis of regulatory issues and options in long-term care. In: Porter VL, Rubin F, eds. *Reform and Regulation in Long-Term Care.* New York: Praeger.
Rawls J (1971). *A Theory of Justice.* Cambridge: Harvard University Press.
Rosenberg, CE (1987). *The Care of Strangers.* New York: Basic Books.
Rothman DJ (1971). *The Discovery of the Asylum: Social Order and Disorder in the New Republic.* Boston: Little, Brown and Co.
Sartorius R (1983). *Paternalism.* Minneapolis: University of Minnesota Press.
Schutz A (1967). *The Phenomenology of the Social World.* Wild J, ed. Evanston, IL: Northwestern University Press.
Seigler M (1982). Confidentiality in medicine: A decrepit concept. *NEJM.* 307: 1518–1521.

Sheild RR (1988). *Uneasy Endings: Daily Life in an American Nursing Home.* Beverly Hills, CA: Sage.

Thomasma DC (1984). Freedom, dependency, and the care of the very old. *J Am Geri Soc.* 32:906–913.

Troeltsch E (1958). *The Social Teachings of the Christian Churches,* 2 vols. New York: Allen Unwin.

Uhlenberg P (1987). A demographic perspective on aging. Chapter 9. *The Elderly as Modern Pioneers.* Bloomington IN: Indiana University Press. 183–205.

Vladeck BC (1980). *Unloving Care: The Nursing Home Tragedy.* New York: Basic Books.

Walters L (1981). The principle of medical confidentiality. In: Mappes TA, Zembaty JS, eds. *Biomedical Ethics.* New York: McGraw-Hill.

Watson G. Free Agency (1975). *J Phil.* 72:205–220.

Watson G. Free Action and Free Will (1987). *Mind.* 96:145–172.

Whitbeck C (1985). Why the attention to paternalism in medical ethics. *J Health Politics, Policy Law.* 10:184–187.

Wolfe DB (1989). Hospitality, health care hybrid shows marketing promise. *Maturity Market Perspectives.* (Nov/Dec):1, 10.

Wolff RP (1970). *In Defense of Anarchism.* New York: Harper & Row.

Zerubavel E (1979). *Patterns of Time in Hospital Life: A Sociological Perspective.* Chicago IL: University of Chicago Press.

Zerubavel E (1981). *Hidden Rhythms: Schedules and Calendars in Social Life.* Chicago IL: University of Chicago Press.

Index